Healing
Joints and Nerves

Immune Stimulation and the New
Science of Regenerative Therapies

Thomas E. Buchheit, MD

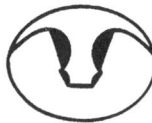

Bull Publishing Company
Boulder, Colorado

Bull Publishing Company
P.O. Box 1377
Boulder, CO 80306
Phone: 800-676-2855
www.bullpub.com

Library of Congress Cataloging-in-Publication Data

Buchheit, Thomas E., author.
   Title: Healing Joints and Nerves / Thomas E. Buchheit.

ISBN 978-1-945188-55-8 (paperback)
Includes bibliographical references and index.

CIP data application in process. Please contact the publisher for further information.

Printed in the USA

29 28 27 26 25   10 9 8 7 6 5 4 3 2 1

Design and production by Dovetail Publishing Services
Cover design by Shannon Bodie, Lightbourne Images

I dedicate this book to Dr. Bill Maixner, a friend and mentor to a generation of researchers, clinicians, and curious individuals. Bill possessed the extraordinary gifts of a sharp mind, a gentle soul, and a tireless work ethic. His spirit lives on in everyone fortunate enough to have known and worked with him. His inspiration and guidance helped launch this book and my six-year writing journey.

Contents

Preface

Why This Book?

Over the years, patients have asked me the most wonderful questions: Are anti-inflammatory medications and steroids harmful? Is osteoarthritis (OA) a result of wear and tear? Is nerve injury irreversible? How does platelet-rich plasma (PRP) work? Do stem cells regenerate new cartilage? How is autologous conditioned serum (ACS) different from platelet-rich plasma? What are exosomes?

I've spent the last two decades seeking answers to these questions. During that time, I realized that most treatments for osteoarthritis and nerve pain do not address the underlying problem, and some may even do more harm than good. Finding solutions felt urgent. I pursued answers by working with top scientists at Duke University, mentoring with a pioneer of regenerative medicine in Düsseldorf, Germany, and scouring through over 1,000 scientific papers. In my studies, all roads led back to the same place: the immune system. The immune cells that heal the body after a cut, sprain, or fracture are the same ones that can be harnessed through regenerative therapies such as platelet-rich plasma, stem cells, and autologous conditioned serum.

One of the challenges of regenerative medicine is the incredible diversity (and confusion) surrounding treatment names, modes of interventions, and sometimes promises of cures. How can someone with osteoarthritis or nerve pain navigate through this fog of information and potential misinformation? The answer again lies in the immune system. Viewing regenerative therapies through the lens of the healing cascade and immune cells offers clarity and comprehension. In this book, I take the reader on the same learning journey I started years ago. As a reader, you will learn what the healing cascade is and how to restart it if it becomes stalled. You'll understand more about the key role exercise, fats, and foods play in providing the essential raw materials needed to resolve chronic inflammation. Finally, you'll recognize how regenerative therapies can jump-start immune cells and alleviate pain. There will be surprises along the way and a few myths debunked. By the end of the book, you'll have a deep understanding of the rapidly evolving field of regenerative medicine. Furthermore, you'll possess the knowledge to evaluate future treatments as they emerge, distinguishing those with promise from those based on flimsy science.

If you're a reader like me, you may occasionally be tempted to skip ahead to chapters of particular personal interest. Try to resist this urge. Your understanding of how the regenerative therapies actually work will be richer if you discover them within the framework of the book's initial foundational chapters. Through this process—of reading from the beginning to the end—you'll understand the science of regenerative medicine.

The medical community is at a watershed moment in treating painful conditions such as osteoarthritis and neuropathy. As you'll learn in this book, the solution isn't to fight inflammation. The solution is to stimulate your body's immune system and harness your built-in healing mechanisms to resolve it. With this book, I hope to provide you, your family, and your friends the tools to heal joints and nerves, reduce pain, and restore function. Enjoy your journey.

Be well,

Tom

Acknowledgments

I would like to give special thanks to Dr. Peter Wehling, a colleague, friend, and pioneer in the fields of regenerative medicine and autobiologics. Peter, thank you for teaching me the nuances, the science, and the power of regenerative therapies, such as autologous conditioned serum.

I want to thank the many individuals who have supported and encouraged me over the years. Dr. Michael Tytell honored me by teaching the intricacies of neurobiology at Wake Forest University and the Marine Biological Laboratory in Woods Hole, Massachusetts. Dr. Richard Rauck educated me on spine interventions and taught me the skills needed to run a clinic. Dr. Jonathan Mark guided me as I transitioned from private practice to academia 15 years ago. Dr. Joseph Mathew supported a fledgling biologics program and consistently kept his word. Dr. Julio Reinecke taught me about the complexities of cytokines, growth factors, and exosomes. Nina Breidenbach patiently showed me proper laboratory techniques, how to work under a hood, and the subtleties of processing ACS. Dr. Jianguo Cheng taught me about MSCs, nerves, and immune involvement in neuropathic pain. Finally, Dr. Luda Diatchenko helped me understand the crucial, paradigm-shifting moment we now experience and the importance of challenging dogma. To these individuals, and many others, I give thanks.

To Dr. Ru-Rong Ji, Thank you for showing me the mechanisms and mysteries behind MSCs and ACS. Over the past decade, I've learned immensely from my time in your laboratory and through our collaborative writing projects.

To Dr. Thomas Van de Ven. Thank you for being a close friend and colleague for the past 15 years. You are a rare individual who can conduct the science while simultaneously demystifying it. Your patience, thoughtfulness, and support have been invaluable.

To Emily Van de Ven, who generously reviewed and assisted me with the initial (and quite dry) book chapters. You helped me find my narrative voice and understand the significant difference between writing a grant application and a book for a broad audience.

To Erin Mulligan, my editor, who continuously pushed me to keep the reader in focus with every word, concept, and paragraph. Your advice was sage. Thank you.

To Jim Bull, my publisher, who took a risk on an author who was not a famous celebrity or influencer. You gave me a chance to explain the wonderful world of regenerative therapies and the intricacies of the immune system. I am immensely grateful and hope this book reaches the diverse audience we envisioned.

To Scott Graham, my friend for over 35 years. Our sub-zero Hok skiing adventures in Quebec and discussions about flavonoids clarified my thinking and helped me construct a challenging chapter. Thank you for your friendship and support throughout these years.

To my parents, Ed and Sandy, who provided unwavering support as I pursued educational and training opportunities, sometimes from a distance. Your sacrifices for your children were generous and often unacknowledged. Belatedly and wholeheartedly, I thank you.

To my children, Sophie, Wade, and Lucas: I thank you for the richness of life you've created for me. I'm so heartened to have watched you all develop into the thoughtful, kind, and focused young adults you have become. Continue to follow your compasses.

To my siblings, Michael, James, and Kristin. You have provided me with strength during important times, career transitions, and life choices. Thank you for always being there.

Most importantly, I want to express my special appreciation to my wife, Kori. Your constant encouragement and support have helped me bring this book from concept to reality. Your love has transformed this labor of love into reality.

Chapter 1

Joint Anatomy and the Myth of "Wear and Tear"

Sarah had studied the basketball game film all week so she could recognize the opposing team's unfolding play. Their star shooter would receive a screen from the center, shake her defender, and dash to the corner for a wide-open jump shot. Anticipating the corner pass, Sarah sprang into action. She lunged forward, her fingertips grazing the ball just enough to knock it loose. It sailed down the court, and Sarah was off—a full sprint toward the basket with her adrenaline drowning out the crowd's roar. Only one defender now stood between her and the basket. As she went up, shifting the ball to her left hand and extending her arm, her torso collided with the defender. She returned to the ground, off balance, her left knee twisted, and she felt a sickening "pop." Sarah crumpled to the floor, and the crowd fell silent. As her teammates helped her off the court, she realized her season had just ended.

Three weeks later, Sarah had anterior cruciate ligament (ACL) surgery. Her recovery took time. She worked intensively with a physical therapist. Physical therapy (PT) can be an invaluable tool. Over months, Sarah regained full knee flexion and rebuilt the strength in her shrunken muscles. Her hard work paid off, and she returned to the team for her senior season. Sarah had a good year, and, importantly, she finished without additional injury. She had some left knee pain and swelling after games, but ice helped and never kept her from giving 100 percent on the court.

In college, Sarah played basketball less often, exchanging this sport for jogging and tennis. She found running a great stress reliever and enjoyed the mental focus that tennis required. She experienced occasional knee stiffness with sports, but it rarely slowed her down. After finishing her economics degree, she moved to the city to work with a respected firm. Sports became not only stress relief but social glue, allowing Sarah to develop new friendships. She ran with a group after work during the week and played in a local tennis league on weekends.

In her 40s, Sarah began to notice pain and swelling in her knee after a tennis match or a longer run. She usually brushed it off. It was nothing compared to the swelling she had after her ACL tear. Ibuprofen seemed to relieve the symptoms, although occasionally it upset her stomach. Unfortunately, over the next few years, her pain began to occur earlier and earlier in her exercise sessions. She thought perhaps she was "overdoing it." She didn't want to quit playing tennis, so she cut back on her running to avoid additional "wear and tear" on her knee.

Cutting back didn't help. The knee pain increased and occurred even when she wasn't playing a sport. Sarah went to see her primary care physician, who ordered X-rays. The X-rays showed moderate osteoarthritis (OA) in her knee with the ACL repair. Her doctor recommended that she start physical therapy and gave her a prescription for the nonsteroidal anti-inflammatory drug (NSAID) celecoxib (Celebrex), hoping it would be less irritating to her stomach than ibuprofen. She found that if she took the medication before playing tennis, she could play longer and have less pain afterward. However, after five or six months, Sarah began to experience some indigestion when taking the celecoxib as well. Her physician told her to decrease the medication as much as possible and gave her a stomach-acid blocker. Sarah cut back on celecoxib, and her knee pain worsened. Frustration set in.

Sarah then made an appointment to see an orthopedic surgeon, hoping a procedure could reduce the pain. The surgeon ordered an MRI that showed her ACL repair was still intact, but the repair was now surrounded by areas of cartilage damage. Sarah and the surgeon talked about knee replacement surgery, but he told her that she was too young. She was only in her 50s, and her activities, over time, might wear out an artificial knee. He offered to inject a steroid into her knee, which she gladly accepted. The particular type of steroid he administered was a corticosteroid. Corticosteroids are different from the many other steroids in the body, including steroid hormones such as testosterone and estrogen. Corticosteroids are produced in the adrenal gland, an organ that sits on top of our kidneys. They suppress inflammation and work with the steroid hormones to control the body's development, metabolism, and response to stress. When someone has a steroid injection for pain, they are typically receiving a corticosteroid. (In this book, I use the common phrase "steroid injection" interchangeably with the more formal term "corticosteroid.")

After Sarah's steroid injection, nearly all her pain disappeared—at least for a while. Unfortunately, after a couple of months, the familiar aches returned. She tried a second steroid injection, but it didn't work as well as the first. Sarah began to pull back from tennis. Her fitness decreased, her weight increased, and her social circle shrank. She had entered orthopedic limbo. In limbo, she experienced pain that prevented her from doing the activities that she loved, and surgery was not an option. She grew resigned, "I guess I'll just need to wait until I can get my knee replaced to get back in shape."

Sarah's story is all too familiar. She was not only in orthopedic limbo without a good pain-relieving option in sight, but she was also afraid to exercise for fear of worsening the wear and tear on her knee. Her beliefs were based on a deeply ingrained theory that weight-loading exercise stresses joints and causes chronic inflammation and cartilage damage. The assumption of Sarah and many others like her is that if a person has painful osteoarthritis, they should reduce impact sports and take nonsteroidal anti-inflammatory drugs like ibuprofen or celecoxib to slow down the inflammation-driven degeneration. Those assumptions might be logical, but they're wrong.

Osteoarthritis: An Antiquated Diagnosis

To understand why the theory of wear and tear evolved and how to better treat osteoarthritis, it is necessary to return to the 1950s. Before the personal computer, before the birth control pill, and before humans landed on the Moon, the system to diagnose OA was developed, and members of the medical community are still using it today. If X-rays (Figure 1.1) show any narrowing of the joint space or small bone spurs, then the medical community designates it as Grade 1 OA, minimal (a). If there is mild joint space narrowing and a definite bone spur, it is Grade 2 OA, mild (b). If there is clear joint space narrowing and more prominent bone spurs, then it is Grade 3 OA, moderate (c). If the joint space is gone and the bone sitting is on bone, it is Grade 4, severe OA (d). The diagnosis of OA hasn't changed in 70 years.

Although this grading system assesses the cushioning space between the bones, it indicates little about the health of the

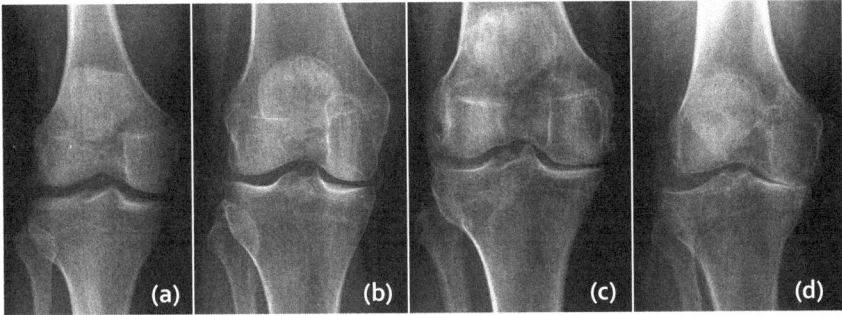

Figure 1.1. Diagnosis of osteoarthritis: X-rays show the progression of osteoarthritis from Grade 1 OA, minimal joint space, narrowing to Grade 4, bone-on-bone appearance with bone spurs.
(© Automatic Grading of Knee Osteoarthritis from Plain Radiographs Using Densely Connected Convolutional Networks).

cartilage, tendons, ligaments, and other factors that drive OA. In this system, the severity of OA is simply assessed like car brake pads that wear over time. The forces that drive that wear are neither addressed nor understood.

Cartilage: A Slippery Surface

To be able to walk, run, bike, or play a sport, people need their joints to move without resistance. This easy motion relies on a smooth, hard, resilient surface created by a specialized tissue called hyaline cartilage. Cartilage cells (chondrocytes) produce hyaline cartilage, an extraordinary substance that tolerates repeated heavy loads and impact forces over our lifetimes. Hyaline cartilage provides these benefits by mixing long strands of tough collagen protein with giant cushioning molecules called proteoglycans (Figure 1.2 on page 6). Proteoglycan molecules contain hyaluronic acid (HA), a large molecule found throughout the body (and in many skin moisturizers). Hyaluronic acid

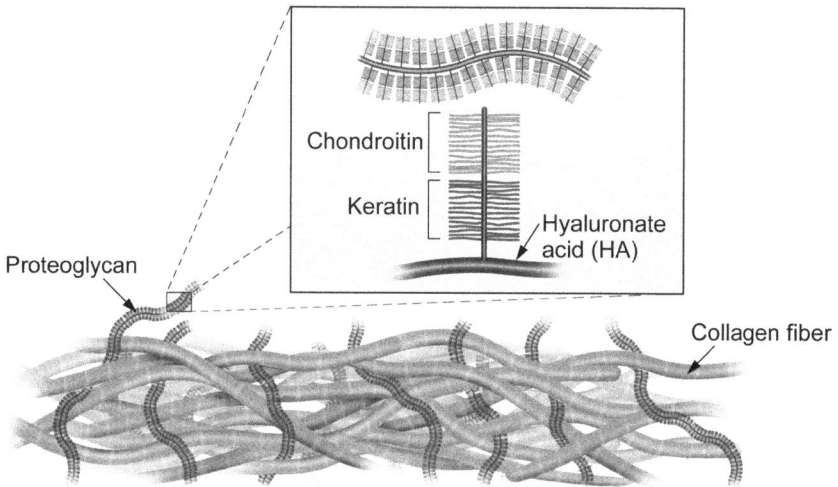

Figure 1.2. Components of hyaline cartilage: Hyaline cartilage gains its strength from collagen woven with proteoglycan molecules. Proteoglycan comprises hyaluronic acid connected to large carbohydrates such as chondroitin and keratin.

provides fullness to the skin and lubrication to the joints. Proteoglycan also contains large carbohydrates, such as keratin and chondroitin. You may be familiar with carbohydrates as a source of energy in your food. Carbohydrates are structures of carbon and water that form sugars such as glucose, which fuel cells and provide a wonderful sweetness in desserts. Carbohydrates, when chained together in long strings, can also provide tremendous structural support. Two of these long carbohydrate chains—keratin and chondroitin—provide the cushion to proteoglycan. They also hold water tightly, increasing the structure's effectiveness as a shock absorber. The giant proteoglycan assembly, with its hyaluronic acid, carbohydrates, and water, provides padding to help joints bounce back after a run, jump, or fall. This padding, combined with the tough collagen fibers, gives hyaline cartilage extraordinary qualities of toughness, smoothness, and resiliency.

The health of hyaline cartilage depends on the activities of the cells that make it—the chondrocytes. As people age, these chondrocytes still produce proteoglycan and other cartilage components, but the cells get sluggish.[1] The quality of the products from chondrocytes also decreases. Fortunately, these chondrocytes respond to stimulation such as exercise. Exercise wakes up the cells and strengthens them. It improves the cells' ability to produce proteoglycan and other building blocks of hyaline cartilage. Contrary to Sarah's belief, walking, jogging, and other weight-bearing exercises *do not* wear away cartilage. These activities improve the health of cartilage by stimulating chondrocytes to produce more robust components for the joint surface. In Chapter 8, Exercise, Inflammation, and Joint Healing, I'll discuss more about how this process occurs.

The hyaline cartilage of the knee also benefits by being tucked within a suction cup rim of softer cartilage called the meniscus (plural: menisci). This softer cartilage, called fibrocartilage, doesn't need to sustain the heavy impacts of its hyaline cartilage cousin. Instead, the fibrocartilage's role is to mold itself around the bones and cradle the joint throughout its range of motion. You can appreciate the flexibility of fibrocartilage by bending the top part of your ear (the pinna), where this flexible cartilage also exists. Fibrocartilage flexes and then snaps back into its usual shape. In the knee, this fibrocartilage is called the meniscus. In the shoulder or hip, it is called the labrum. The menisci and labrums serve the same purpose. They keep joints aligned when people walk, run, or throw objects. The fibrocartilage also helps to evenly distribute the forces of impact on a joint. When you land from a jump, the meniscus softens the blow to the hyaline cartilage. Through these activities, fibrocartilage is tremendously protective of joints and the hyaline cartilage surfaces.

The importance of the knee meniscus hasn't always been appreciated. As recently as the 1980s, it was common for patients with a meniscus injury to have this fibrocartilage completely removed—an operation called a meniscectomy. At the time, surgeons believed the knee was better off with no meniscus than a damaged one. Although well-intentioned, this surgical procedure actually *increased* the patient's chances of later developing knee osteoarthritis.[2] Without a meniscus, abnormal motion, low-level damage, and chronic inflammation in the knee are much more likely to occur. Many of the individuals who had a surgical meniscus removal in the 1980s and 1990s ended up with a knee replacement surgery a few years later. These individuals would have been better off with intensive physical therapy and strengthening exercises to protect the knee joint. The more stable the motion of a joint is, the more it is protected from OA.

Tendons and Ligaments: Holding Us Together

Tendons, ligaments, and muscles form the external support system of a joint. Tendons connect muscle to bone. Ligaments connect bone to bone. Muscles do the work. Together, these structures stabilize joints and ensure that your parts move in specific and reliable directions (Figure 1.3). As muscles contract, allowing you to walk, run, or throw objects, the force transmits through your tendons to your bone anchors. The tension these structures carry is tremendous. For instance, the tension on the quadriceps tendon (connecting the quadriceps muscles to the patella) and the patellar tendon (continuing that connection to the lower tibia bone) can be three to four times your body weight when landing from a jump. Tendons, like cartilage, have collagen and proteoglycan. Tendons also feature

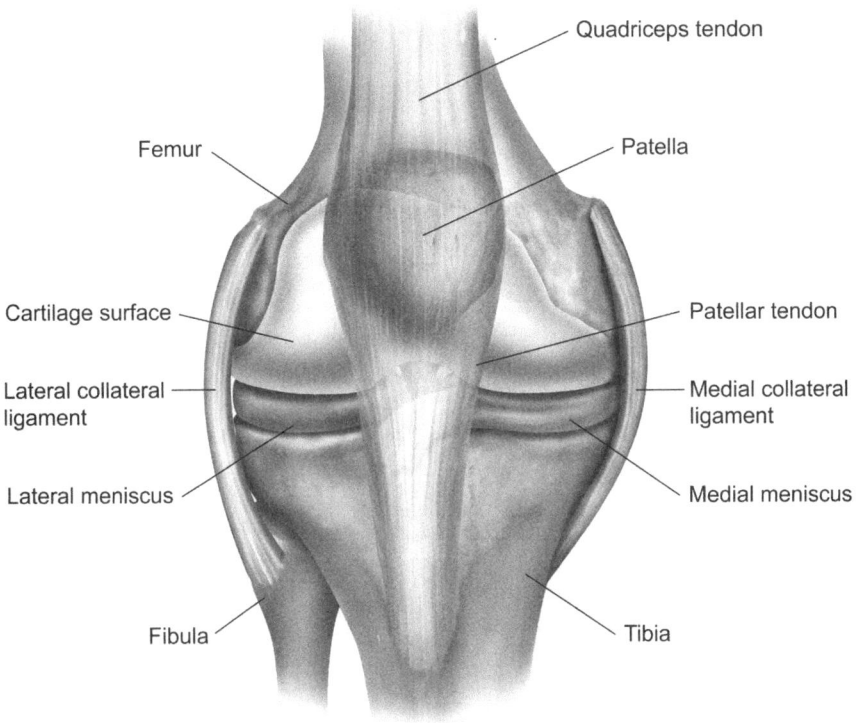

Figure 1.3. Meniscus, tendons, and ligaments of the knee: The medial and lateral menisci are fibrocartilage structures that stabilize the knee during motion and cushion impact. The quadriceps and patellar tendons connect the quadriceps thigh muscles to the tibia. The medial and lateral collateral ligaments provide side-to-side stability.

long, flexible proteins called elastin that help to buffer forces as they are transmitted to bone. Elastin adds protection from injury with jumps, falls, or other extraordinary forces. Tendons are remarkably resilient. Nonetheless, when forces are extreme or applied repetitively without recovery time, tendon damage can occur. About 30 percent of sports injuries are attributed to tendon damage.[3]

Historically, physicians called any damage to a tendon "tendonitis" (the suffix "itis" implies inflammation). Although still commonly used, the term tendonitis increasingly falls out of favor as the medical community continues to understand more about these vital structures. Portable ultrasound, which has become almost ubiquitous in sports and musculoskeletal clinics, has given clarity and insight into tendon anatomy. Ultrasound now allows medical professionals to distinguish between inflammation of a tendon and chronic, nonhealing degeneration. Often, when evaluating patients with shoulder pain, I'll see deterioration of the rotator cuff tendons on ultrasound but no inflammation. These people have a tendinopathy, not tendonitis. The suffix "pathy" means disease in general, with or without inflammation. While this distinction may seem overly academic if you're suffering from shoulder pain, it allows the treating physician to focus on therapies that promote long-term healing. If physicians and patients focus only on suppressing inflammation when there isn't much inflammation present, it's unlikely to do the patient long-term good.

Just as cartilage has its embedded cells called chondrocytes, tendons have cells called tenocytes. These tenocytes produce collagen, proteoglycan, elastin, and the other materials that make up the structure of the tendon—the tendon's matrix.[4] Like cartilage, tenocyte activity and matrix production can be stimulated by exercise, responding best to activities that put some stress on the tendon. In other words, moderate strain induces healing, but excessive strain too soon after an injury can worsen damage.[5]

For example, an exercise that physical therapists use for Achilles tendinopathy of the ankle is called a "heel raise." In this activity, you raise yourself up on your tiptoes and then slowly drop your heels back to the floor. This exercise puts the weight of your body on the Achilles tendon, straining it and stimulating the tenocytes to begin their repair work. However, if you did a hundred heel raises on day one of your exercise program for your

Achilles pain, you would probably further damage the tendons. The key is moderation. Physical therapists are skilled in knowing where this "Goldilocks" position is. They can help a client develop an exercise regime to optimize tendon health not only at the Achilles but also the rotator cuff of the shoulder, the patellar tendon of the knee, gluteal tendons of the hip, and other structures prone to injury.

Ligaments share many structural similarities with tendons. However, a tendon connects muscle to bone, but a ligament connects bone to bone. Ligaments stabilize and protect joints throughout defined ranges of motion. For instance, the ligaments on the inside and outside of the knee (the medial and lateral collateral ligaments) provide crucial side-to-side stability, especially when you are playing sports (Figure 1.3). Ligaments and tendons also share a unique characteristic. They sense pain. Whereas cartilage has no nerve supply and, therefore, can't feel pain, ligaments and tendons have rich nerve supplies. The nerve supply grows and sensitizes after an injury. If you've ever experienced a ligament or tendon tear, you likely became quickly aware of their rich nerve supply.

Understanding the nerve supply to joints also provides insight into osteoarthritis pain. Since cartilage has no nerves and no sensation, osteoarthritis pain is from structures in and around the joint: the bones, ligaments, and tendons. So, if an individual is experiencing pain with OA, it's not from the structure that an X-ray monitors—the cartilage; it's the rest of the joint that is giving them problems.

Not only can injured tendons and ligaments become painful themselves, but they can also cause inflammation in a nearby bursa. Bursa are fluid-filled sacs that offer cushion from adjacent bone or other areas of potential abrasion. Common locations for bursitis include the shoulder (around the rotator cuff tendons) and the side of the hip (around the gluteal tendons). Bursitis, in combination with tendinopathy, is quite common. In cases where a person has both, the bursa and the tendon must be treated individually for long-term benefit. When a corticosteroid is used to treat bursitis, distinguishing the bursa from the nearby tendon is essential. The same corticosteroid used to decrease bursa inflammation may be damaging to the tendons. There have even been reports of tendon ruptures after being injected with a steroid. Before the use of ultrasound, medical professionals had to rely on anatomic guides to perform injections. In the shoulder, studies show that physicians and surgeons likely missed the target up to 30 percent of the time.[6] Ultrasound guidance has provided a leap forward in accuracy and safety.

Your joints are not static pieces of hardware but dynamic, remarkable structures capable of repair and recovery. Cartilage, tendons, and ligaments contain living cells that can be activated with exercise to generate healthy new building blocks. Sarah's exercise program was not "wear and tear" for her joints. Her osteoarthritis was caused by her ACL injury with prolonged and unchecked inflammation in her knee, not from the activities she enjoyed in adulthood.

The next chapter discusses how inflammation, proteins called cytokines, and enzymes are responsible for Sarah's joint damage and OA.

Takeaways

1. Osteoarthritis is not a "wear and tear" disease.
2. Joint cartilage benefits from strong support structures, including the meniscus, tendons, and ligaments.
3. Tendon damage without inflammation (tendinopathy) is common.

Chapter 2

How to Damage Cartilage: Cytokines and Enzymes

Sarah received a steroid injection for her knee osteoarthritis, which temporarily relieved her pain. The injection didn't change the cartilage space between her bones or on her X-rays. It altered the immune state of her knee by suppressing certain types of cytokines. It was the cytokines that determined the severity of Sarah's pain. It was also cytokines that triggered the development of her OA.

Cytokines: Immune Cell Messengers

Each of the major joints (knee, hip, shoulder) is surrounded by a joint capsule called the synovium. Synovial cells line the capsule and produce the joint fluid and proteins that bathe the moving surfaces. Immune cells in the capsule secrete cytokines that drive or resolve chronic inflammation depending on the types and amounts secreted. In future chapters, I'll describe the specific kinds of immune cells responsible for inflammation and recovery. For now, I will focus on the cytokine proteins these immune cells produce and the effects of these cytokines on cartilage.

Cytokines have a poor reputation. They are responsible for significant pain in chronic inflammatory and autoimmune conditions. In autoimmune diseases, such as rheumatoid arthritis (RA) or Crohn's disease, the body reacts against itself, sometimes producing massive concentrations of inflammatory cytokines. In RA, this causes pain, swelling, and joint damage. In Crohn's disease, it causes inflammation of the intestines with subsequent pain, diarrhea, and even breakdown of the intestinal wall. Cytokines also produce the aches and pains of the flu, worsen sepsis with bacterial infections, and cause lung damage with COVID-19. Despite their negative reputation, cytokines aren't always harmful. Cytokines are a broad spectrum of proteins that regulate all aspects of immune function, good and bad. Without them, people would struggle to defend against bacterial or viral infection, fight off cancer cells, or grow stronger with exercise.

Tumor Necrosis Factor: Friend or Foe?

There are several families of cytokines proteins, including tumor necrosis factor (TNF), interleukins, and interferons. TNF was one of the earlier cytokines identified. In the late 1800s, a cancer surgeon named Dr. William Coley was practicing at the New York Memorial Hospital, where he struggled to treat cancers without modern-day chemotherapy agents. He became fascinated with the story of a patient with a recurrent facial tumor. The patient had undergone several surgeries, only to have the cancer reoccur. On the final surgery, the mass could not be removed entirely, and the wound became infected. This was a common occurrence in the days before antibiotics. But, with each bout of fever from the infection, the tumor appeared to shrink. Over several months and several rounds of fevers, the cancer completely disappeared. Curious about the long-term outcome, Dr. Coley tracked the patient down several years later. The patient remained cancer-free. It appeared that the immune system's response to infection had cured his tumor.

Dr. Coley tried to reproduce this anticancer effect in several patients by intentionally infecting their tumors with bacteria. Sometimes it worked. Sometimes it didn't. Sometimes the infection proved fatal. He then switched to an inoculation with dead bacterial parts, now referred to as "Coley's Toxins." These toxins produced a strong immune stimulus and reduced the risk of death from infection. He went on to treat hundreds of cancer patients with his "toxins." Many of these treatments were remarkably successful in patients who had few alternatives. But with Coley's death in 1936, significant skepticism from the medical community, and the development of chemotherapy agents, the use of Coley's Toxins in the treatment of cancers largely disappeared.

In the 1970s at the same hospital, now called Memorial Sloan-Kettering Cancer Center, Dr. Lloyd Old and researcher Elizabeth Carswell revived the concept of using infection to treat cancer. These researchers started treating mouse tumors with an injection of weakened bacteria. Like Dr. Coley, they saw regression and sometimes the extraordinary disappearance of the cancers. Carswell and Old had access to laboratory techniques not available in the late 1800s. They were able to track the types and concentrations of proteins secreted after the mice were infected (and sometimes cured). In 1975, they published their findings of an immune cell protein—a cytokine—responsible for the anti-tumor effects. Since this cytokine protein could necrose (kill) tumors, they named it tumor necrosis factor (TNF).[1]

Carswell and Old's positive research results generated enthusiasm for TNF as a potential cancer therapy in humans. Unfortunately, when tested in patients, TNF appeared to be more effective in making patients ill than killing their tumors. Although TNF is still considered an option in rare cases where it can be directly infused into the tumor, the therapy has largely been abandoned because of pain, inflammation, and other side effects.[2]

Even though TNF never became widely used to treat cancer, the work of Carswell and Old in identifying the cytokine protein led to other discoveries. TNF proteins were found in high concentrations in the joints of patients with RA and the intestines of those with Crohn's disease. These discoveries prompted scientists to ask the next logical question: If TNF is elevated in diseases such as RA, would suppressing TNF treat those disorders?

Designing a drug to turn off TNF wasn't easy. To suppress this cytokine without significant side effects required focused and accurate targeting. Researchers looked to antibodies. Antibodies are masters at finding and locking to specific proteins. This skill is how they help people fight bacteria and viruses. Antibodies recognize and bind tightly to proteins on the surface of the invading bacteria or virus, neutralizing and ultimately destroying it. Antibody-based drugs would confer a similar accurate targeting of the TNF protein. Since antibodies are created by the immune system of a living organism, an antibody-based drug needs to be biologically, not synthetically, manufactured. In the case of the first TNF inhibitor, mouse cells were used to make it.

The first antibody-based TNF blocker was tested in patients with refractory RA—that is, RA that doesn't respond to standard treatments. The results were promising. Patients had decreased pain, joint swelling, fatigue, and inflammation in the body.[3] More extensive follow-up studies confirmed these results, and the first biologically manufactured drug to suppress TNF called etanercept (Enbrel) was approved in 1998. Several others soon followed, including infliximab (Remicade) and adalimumab (Humira). These drugs frequently have an "ab" at the end of their name, signifying that they are antibody based and target a specific protein or molecule. The use of TNF inhibitors has been of enormous benefit to those with RA and other autoimmune and inflammatory conditions.

Interleukins: Cytokines with Many Functions

Interleukins (IL) acquired their name when they were discovered as messengers between white blood cells (leukocytes). Interleukins control immune activation and help us fight viral and bacterial invaders (Figure 2.1 on page 18). These immune proteins can also cause significant inflammation, pain, and tissue destruction if released for prolonged periods. Interleukin-1 (IL-1) is produced by several types of leukocytes, such as the macrophage, which I'll discuss in future chapters. IL-1 is one of the most destructive or catabolic cytokines for cartilage. Catabolic comes from the Greek word *katabole*, which means to throw down. Even small doses of IL-1, the catabolic cytokine, can produce significant arthritic changes within a joint. There are several biologically manufactured inhibitors of IL-1 that are used to treat rheumatoid arthritis and other autoimmune conditions.

Interleukin-6 (IL-6) is a cytokine with multiple and diverse effects. IL-6 is elevated in the joints of people with rheumatoid arthritis and can cause significant lung and blood vessel damage in individuals with COVID-19. Chronically elevated IL-6 levels, like IL-1, produce damage to joint tissues and cartilage. Several IL-6 blockers have also been developed to treat the excessive concentrations of the cytokine IL-6 in RA. IL-6

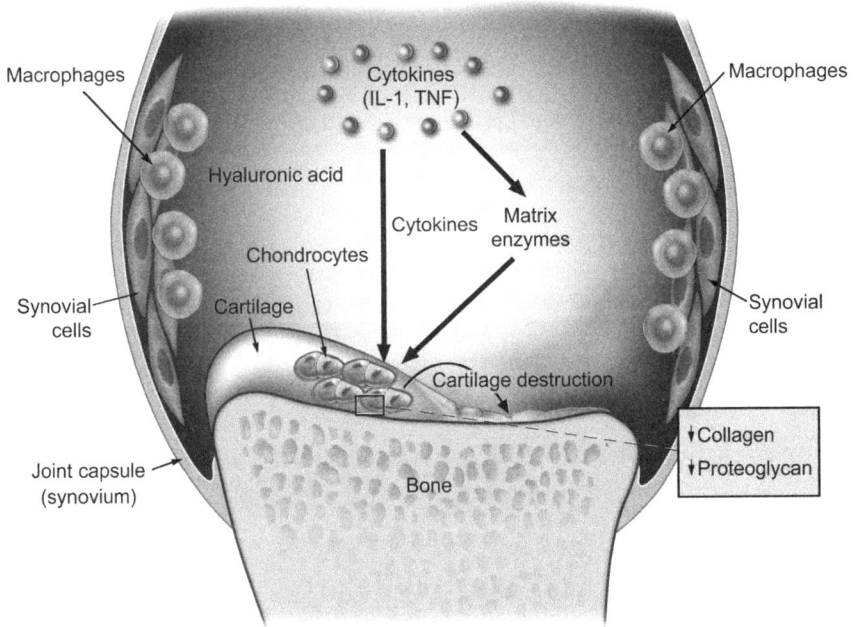

Figure 2.1. The causes of osteoarthritis: Hyaluronic acid and other lubricating proteins are made by the synovial cells of the joint capsule. Inflammatory cytokines from leukocytes (such as the macrophage) trigger matrix enzymes to split hyaluronic acid into smaller inflammatory pieces and break down cartilage. The broken-down hyaluronic acid fragments further increase the release of inflammatory cytokines in a vicious feedback cycle.

inhibitors are often used when other cytokine blockers are ineffective.

IL-6 can also play some beneficial roles, such as in exercise. IL-6 is significantly increased with a workout, a topic I'll explore in Chapter 8, Exercise, Inflammation, and Joint Healing. Because IL-6 is thought to be necessary to produce strength gains with exercise, some sports scientists call IL-6 an exerkine to distinguish this positive role from the damaging role it may play in RA or other diseases.

Interferons: Fighting Viruses

Interferons are a third major class of cytokines. These cytokines are called interferons because they interfere with virus function and help fight the infection. You've probably experienced the effects of these potent immune stimulators. The fever, aches, and chills you experience with the flu are partially due to interferons. Interferons also act as communication proteins between immune cells and nerves. The crosstalk between inflammatory immune cells and nerves is one of the drivers of the aches and pains that accompany a viral infection. That ache is a sign that the cytokines are doing their work in fighting the disease.

Enzyme Destruction: The Result of a Cytokine Imbalance

If inflammatory and catabolic cytokines aren't kept in check, they can unleash a host of damaging enzymes. Enzymes, like cytokines, aren't all bad. More than 75,000 of these specialized proteins speed up chemical reactions and are necessary for life. Enzymes help you digest food, build proteins, and provide energy. Without them, your cells would freeze up, unable to carry out their most basic functions. Certain kinds of enzymes can also break down tissues. If exposed to excessive concentrations of inflammatory cytokines, enzymes in the joint called matrix metalloproteinases (MMPs) are produced in large quantities and damage the collagen and proteoglycan of cartilage.

MMP enzymes also cut up lubricating molecules, such as hyaluronic acid (HA), that are produced by the synovial cells of the joint. These HA fragments lose their ability to lubricate the joint and further increase inflammation. This process becomes a vicious feedback cycle: MMP enzymes break down HA and cartilage, which causes more inflammation and produces more enzyme release.[4] Unless cytokine balance is restored, this cycle leads to OA (see Figure 2.1).

Not All Bad News: Some Cytokines Resolve Inflammation

You've now read about several cytokines that can cause intense inflammation. But inflammation is only one aspect of cytokine function. These proteins are equally capable of resolving inflammation and restoring balance. One of these inflammation-resolvers is IL-1Ra, a cytokine that binds to the same receptor as IL-1. It effectively shuts down the inflammatory effects of IL-1. After an injury, immune cells produce IL-1Ra after a few days of inflammation to help with healing. IL-1Ra is considered "anabolic" because of its ability to rebuild and restore tissues. Anabolic, from the Greek *anabole*, means to throw upward and reflects these constructive and restorative actions. The production of IL-1Ra is the body's natural reaction to re-establish balance and tissue health.

Other inflammation-resolving cytokines, such as IL-10, can reduce immune cell production of TNF and interferons. If released in large enough quantities, IL-10, IL-1Ra, and several other inflammation-resolving cytokines can help restore the balance of catabolic (destructive) and anabolic (constructive) forces and improve joint health.

Suppressing Inflammatory Cytokines to Treat Osteoarthritis?

What if naturally produced inflammation-resolving cytokines such as IL-1Ra and IL-10 are not sufficient to restore immune balance and prevent osteoarthritis? In this situation, it might make sense to look to the cytokine-suppressing drugs. If inhibitors of IL-1 or TNF reduce pain and joint damage in RA, and those same cytokines (IL-1 and TNF) are also present in OA, might these suppressor drugs also treat OA? This hypothesis has been tested several times in the past few years. One of the first tests of a cytokine inhibitor for patients with OA was the IL-1 blocker called anakinra. Unfortunately, injections of anakinra were no more effective than injections of a placebo (salt water) in reducing patients' pain and stiffness.[5] Studies were also done with inhibitors of inflammatory TNF. Even patients with OA and evidence of inflammation on MRI didn't experience reductions in pain with these powerful cytokine inhibitors.[6]

These failures surprised many researchers (and me at the time). If patients with OA had evidence of inflammation and increased concentrations of inflammatory cytokines, why didn't blocking these cytokines reduce pain? The reason is that the approach to OA has been oversimplified. Fighting inflammation isn't the answer.

Do X-Rays Tell the Story?

The drivers of osteoarthritis are the immune cells, their cytokines, and the destructive enzymes the cytokines turn on. Yet the diagnosis of OA includes none of these factors. It relies on the X-ray changes of narrowing between the bones. Not surprisingly, there is a poor correlation between the severity of pain and the severity of OA shown on X-ray. One Harvard study of over three hundred individuals with moderate-to-severe knee arthritis on X-ray found that almost half had *no pain*.[7] Similar poor correlations between pain and X-ray findings have also been seen in other joints. Researchers from the UK studied the relationship between hip pain and the severity of OA as shown on X-ray. They found almost no association between individuals with mild to moderate OA X-rays and patient pain. Only X-ray evidence of severe hip OA was correlated with pain.[8] This divergence between pain and X-ray findings is not surprising. X-rays tell us about the past. X-rays tell us that the joint was exposed to damaging cytokines and enzymes (that break down collagen and proteoglycans), and thin cartilage. Pain is created by multiple structures within the joint except for, ironically, the one doctors measure to judge its severity—the cartilage.

The poor correlation between pain and medical images occurs in other body areas and other forms of medical imaging, such as the shoulder. When MRIs became available and popular for diagnosing rotator cuff disease in the 1990s, it was assumed that the severity of rotator cuff tendon tears would also predict the severity of pain. In 1995, orthopedic researchers from the University of Miami challenged this notion. They performed MRIs on the shoulders of approximately one hundred individuals who had no pain. Of those aged 40 to 60, over 25 percent had a rotator cuff tear. In individuals over 60, more than 50 percent had a rotator cuff tear.[9] The presence of a tear did not correlate with the presence of pain, especially in those over 60. The MRI was also reporting on the past.

What about individuals with severe pain but only minimal OA changes on X-ray? Their pain tells us that their immune system is activated and likely releasing inflammatory cytokines and MMP enzymes, regardless of the X-ray images. These patients have the immune imbalance of OA with or without X-ray changes. Individuals with these inflammatory changes are also at greater risk of rapidly losing their cartilage and developing X-ray evidence of OA.[10] Patients with significant pain but only minor X-ray changes of OA would likely benefit from early intervention to halt the process that damages cartilage and tissues. I'll discuss these interventions in later chapters.

The Importance of Balance

Suppressing cytokines and the immune system is not the long-term solution to treat OA. Medical treatment must strive for a balance of these immune proteins and their related enzymes. With balance, treatment can prevent the runaway inflammation and cartilage destruction that leads to OA without losing immune cell activities that guard against infection and repair tissues. Sarah's X-rays showed that she had previously experienced an imbalance of cytokines and MMP enzymes, leading to the breakdown of knee cartilage and the X-ray diagnosis of OA. Her current pain indicates that the immune imbalance is ongoing. She had corticosteroids injected into her knee, temporarily suppressing inflammation and reducing pain. Would repeated steroid injections reduce the inflammation and enzyme damage to her knee?

In the next chapter, I'll present the pros and cons of steroid injections, anti-inflammatory medications, hyaluronic acid injections, and surgery to treat OA. I'll also explain why immune suppression may have unfortunate longer-term effects.

Takeaways

1. Inflammatory cytokines cause pain and increase the enzymes that damage cartilage in OA.
2. Blocking cytokines is not effective in treating OA.
3. X-rays correlate poorly with a patient's OA pain. They tell us about the past, not the present immune state of the joint.

Chapter 3

Current Osteoarthritis Treatments:
Chemistry, Steroids, Hardware

The first medication that Sarah reached for when her knee pain flared was a nonsteroidal anti-inflammatory drug (NSAID). This family of medications, used regularly by over 30 million Americans, originates in ancient civilizations and the bark of a willow tree. Tea from this bark has been used for centuries to treat rheumatic fever and pain. It contains an anti-inflammatory compound called salicylic acid, generally considered the first NSAID. Salicylic acid works similarly to modern NSAIDs by blocking an enzyme called cyclooxygenase (COX). When COX is blocked, the body reduces its production of inflammatory lipids called prostaglandins. Reducing inflammatory prostaglandins reduces pain. But to understand how society moved from willow bark tea to modern NSAIDS that fill pharmacy shelves, it's helpful to first travel back to the late 1800s and the work of a German chemist, Felix Hoffmann.

Chemistry: From Willow Bark to Modern NSAIDs

Hoffmann finished his PhD in Munich, Germany, in 1893 and was offered a position in the research department at Bayer Pharmaceuticals. One of his goals was to find methods to improve the safety and tolerability of analgesics (pain-relieving medications) such as salicylic acid. The willow bark extract was an effective pain reliever but also notorious for its side effects, such as stomach irritation. Hoffmann's father, who suffered from rheumatoid arthritis, knew these side effects firsthand. Hoffmann and the chemistry team at Bayer combined salicylic acid with several different compounds, searching for a way to decrease the toxicity of this anti-inflammatory. Ultimately, they joined it with acetic acid (vinegar), creating *acetyl*salicylic acid. Side effects decreased, and the new synthetic NSAID—aspirin—was launched in 1899 by Bayer and remains one of the most widely used medications on the globe. Approximately 60 billion tablets of acetylsalicylic acid are consumed each year worldwide. Ibuprofen—which, like aspirin, is a COX inhibitor—arrived on US shelves in 1974 and immediately became popular for its effectiveness and relatively low incidence of side effects. Ibuprofen was soon joined by other NSAIDs, including naproxen and diclofenac.

In the late 1990s and early 2000s, a new type of NSAID called a COX-2 inhibitor appeared. Biochemists have known for some time that two different forms of the COX enzymes produce prostaglandin lipids. COX-1 enzymes make prostaglandins that carry out essential "housekeeping" functions in the body, such as kidney blood flow and the production of gastric lining. COX-2 enzymes produce the prostaglandins that cause inflammation, pain, and swelling. Until COX-2 inhibitors were created, the available NSAIDs (including aspirin and ibuprofen) affected both COX-1 and COX-2 pathways. This led to reductions in pain but also complications of stomach ulcers and kidney dysfunction.

To maximize the anti-inflammatory potency and minimize the undesired side effects, pharmaceutical chemists developed several compounds that only inhibited the COX-2 enzyme. Celecoxib (Celebrex) was the first of these, released in 1998, almost exactly a century after the release of aspirin. Cele-coxib was followed by even more selective COX-2 inhibitor drugs such as rofecoxib (Vioxx) in 1999 and valdecoxib (Bextra) in 2001. These medications were considered a significant advancement in pharmacologic precision and safety. Patients loved them, and nearly all physicians (including me) prescribed them. Unfortunately, in 2004, the medical community learned that rofecoxib increased the rate of heart attacks. Rofecoxib was removed from the shelves. Valdecoxib was also soon discontinued. The two less selective COX-2 inhibitors, celecoxib and meloxicam (Mobic), seemed to have fewer cardiac side effects and have remained in use in the US.

Regardless of which enzyme an NSAID inhibits or how selective it is, there is no completely safe NSAID for long-term use. NSAIDs increase the risk of gastrointestinal bleeding and double the chances of kidney injury in individuals over the age of 65. Because of these risks and side effects, I speak with quite a few people who have turned to another analgesic, acetaminophen, for their arthritis pain. Although in high doses, acetaminophen can be toxic to the liver, in modest amounts, it is likely safer than chronic NSAIDs. Unfortunately, for many, acetaminophen is less effective in treating osteoarthritis pain. The issues with these medications can leave patients stuck between a rock and a hard place. Effective, safe, long-term medication options are nearly nonexistent for OA.

Steroids: Cow Adrenals to Synthetics

There are millions of corticosteroid injections performed in the US every year for OA pain that doesn't respond to oral medications. These injections, such as triamcinolone (Kenalog) and methylprednisolone (Depo-Medrol), can provide rapid and dramatic pain relief. I still perform corticosteroid injection procedures because a steroid injection can give patients a window of opportunity for exercise. The injection can help them make functional gains by working out with their physical therapist or trainer. There is also evidence that a single steroid dose can improve cell energy supply and function.[1] But some people cannot make advances despite their best efforts. They find themselves returning for repeated injections, trying to regain that freedom of movement and pain relief that injections briefly afforded them.

The story of steroid injections for arthritis goes back to the 1920s and a physician named Dr. Philip Hench. After finishing his military service, Hench began his fellowship at the Mayo Foundation in 1923, and three years later, he was named the head of the new Department of Rheumatic Diseases. This was likely not an easy position, as treatments for rheumatoid arthritis (RA) and other autoimmune conditions were frustratingly limited. At that time, a patient could look forward to a course of high-dose aspirin, bed rest, and sometimes the injection of gold salts to treat the disease.

In the 1930s, Hench began work with two biochemists, Edward Kendall from the Mayo Clinic and Tadeus Reichstein from Zurich, Switzerland. Hench was seeking new methods to treat the painful, swollen joints of RA patients he was seeing in the clinic. The three scientists began by trying to isolate inflammation-suppressing hormones from the adrenal glands of cows, which was neither easy nor glamorous work. To extract small amounts of compound E, later defined as the corticosteroid cortisol, they needed to process hundreds of pounds of cow adrenals. By 1948, they finally had enough purified adrenal extract to treat a woman suffering from RA. Twice daily injections of compound E into her muscles quickly improved her joint pain, although she also experienced facial puffiness, acne, and "hostile ideation" with the treatment.[2] It's a bit unclear exactly what the researchers meant by hostile ideation, but it was likely the first description of anger and aggression associated with the use of steroids. She probably had the first documented case of "roid rage." It appears that the side effects for her were almost as memorable as the pain relief.

The first injection of these adrenal extracts into a joint was performed in 1950 for the knees of a patient with rheumatoid arthritis.[3] The reductions in pain and swelling were impressive, although short-lived. Repeated injections were required to sustain the results. Nonetheless, the benefits exceeded all other options, and the race to produce more of these valuable corticosteroid compounds began.

By 1952, improved extraction and processing techniques for cortisone were developed. By 1958, six fully synthetic steroids were available for widespread use in treating autoimmune diseases such as RA. Hench, Kendall, and Reichstein shared the 1950 Nobel Prize in Physiology or Medicine. The Nobel committee commended them for their tireless, collaborative work "relating to the hormones of the adrenal cortex, their structure, and biological effects."

Enthusiasm for steroid injections for ailments in addition to rheumatoid arthritis, such as osteoarthritis, ballooned at this time. In 1951, Dr. Joseph Hollander at the University of Pennsylvania published the results of steroid injections for 37 patients with OA, noting that 36 had a "complete or nearly complete disappearance of symptoms." Duration of improvement, however, did not factor into his definition of success. Some of the patients required up to 17 injections per year. Perhaps this is why, despite the apparent successes he reported, Hollander shared a word of caution for steroid injections in OA treatment, noting, "the advisability of using these agents

is doubtful because of expense and possible dangers, particularly in persons past middle age—the very group suffering from
osteoarthritis."[3] The dangers that Dr. Hollander was referring
to were not only the observed "hostile ideation" and aggres-
sive behavior, but also the suppression of the body's own steroid
production after repeated steroid injections.

The body's adrenal glands—small, triangular-shaped glands
located on top of both kidneys—naturally make corticosteroids,
such as cortisol, at different rates depending on the time of day,
stress exposure, and multiple other factors. The production of
cortisol and other hormones in the adrenal glands is regulated
by structures at the base of the brain called the hypothalamus
and pituitary. Together, the hypothalamus, pituitary, and adrenal
glands (HPA axis) function to continuously monitor corticosteroid hormone levels in the body, whether the steroids are made
naturally, injected into a muscle or a joint, or taken orally. When
steroid levels rise, the HPA axis responds by shutting off production to avoid excesses (Figure 3.1). That means that if you're on
oral or injectable steroids for a longer term (weeks to months),
your adrenal production of natural corticosteroids, such as cortisol, goes dormant. This is why you need to do a slow taper when
stopping steroid treatment. The slow decrease allows the HPA
axis to re-activate your body's natural manufacturing processes.

With the dramatic rise of corticosteroids in the treatment of
RA and OA, physicians quickly became aware of the other risks
of repeated injections, including reductions in bone density
and tissue healing. Steroids alter the delicate balance between
bone anabolic (building) and catabolic (breaking down) activities, decreasing bone mineral density and strength.[4] The loss
of bone density can become severe in some individuals (called
osteoporosis), increasing the risk of fracture. At the hip and
spine, these fractures can be devastating.

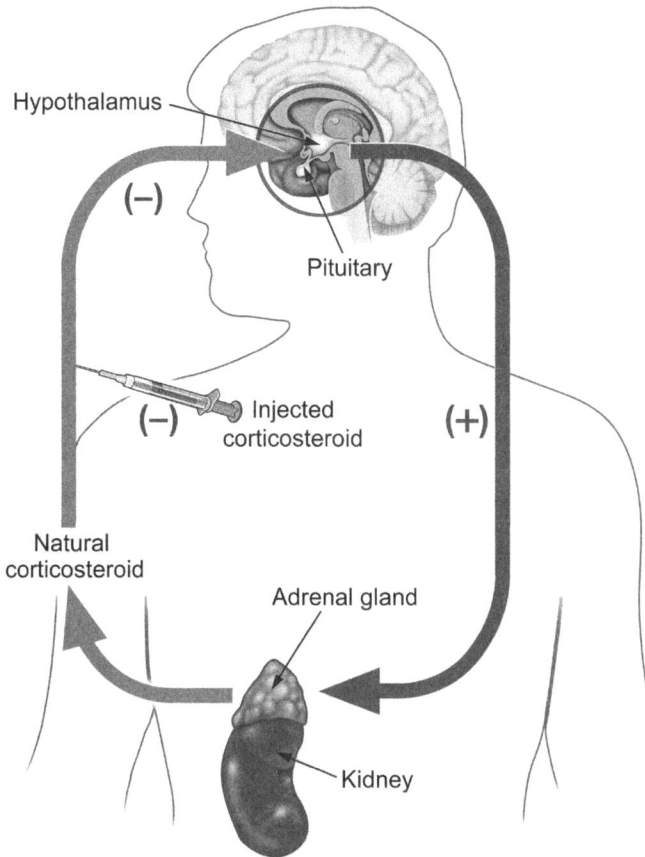

Figure 3.1. The effect of steroid injections on hypothalamus-pituitary-adrenal (HPA) function: Frequent injections of corticosteroids will suppress HPA function, decreasing the body's production of natural steroids such as cortisol.

Chronic steroids also inhibit tissue repair after injury. As part of your immune system, white blood cells circulate in your blood and respond to injury or illness. They migrate to the area of damage and release multiple growth factors that start the healing and repair process. Steroids can inhibit these white blood cell functions and slow down their migration to damaged areas.[5] When this happens, the healing machinery is never fully engaged and wound repair is compromised.

Despite the concerns about bone and immune system side effects with repeated steroid injections, tens of thousands of patients still rely on this procedure to maintain activity. Medication options are too limited and ineffective. In addition to bone and immune system changes, in 2017, the medical community also learned that steroid injections for osteoarthritis may be harming the very joint it is trying to treat. Researchers from Tufts University published the results of a two-year randomized trial of corticosteroid injections for knee osteoarthritis in *The Journal of the American Medical Association.*

In this study, patients received an MRI and either steroid or saline injections every three months. At the end of the study, the participants' pain and knee function were evaluated and they had a repeat MRI. Most physicians who read this publication weren't surprised that the steroid injections didn't provide long-term improvements in pain or function. The disturbing surprise was that the follow-up MRIs showed that those who received the steroids had more significant cartilage damage in their knees than those who received saline.[6] For these patients, shutting down inflammation with repeated corticosteroids didn't slow the development of OA. On the contrary, it sped it up. Although corticosteroids are powerful tools to treat runaway inflammation, frequent dosing comes at a cost.

Hardware: Oil Changes and Joint Replacements

Since the 1990s, injections of hyaluronic acid (HA) have also been used to treat the pain of OA. Recall from Figure 2.1 on page 18 how enzymes such as matrix metalloproteinases (MMP) can break down the large, lubricating HA molecules in the synovial fluid. The smaller fragments of HA lose their ability to lubricate the joint surfaces and worsen chronic inflammation. Therefore, replacing the degraded HA molecules with larger ones should improve joint lubrication and decrease inflammation. Multiple HA products are now available in the United States. Some are from natural sources; others are synthetic. Over the past few decades, numerous studies have shown that HA injections can slightly improve pain, but these improvements are modest. Because of the limited pain relief and higher cost of HA injections (significantly more than a steroid injection), several groups, such as the American Academy of Orthopedic Surgeons and the American College of Rheumatology, have recommend against using HA injections for OA.[7] Despite these recommendations, HA injection is still performed by thousands of physicians and surgeons in the US, including me. The reason is simple: It is still a safer option than chronic medications or repeated steroid injections.

For those with bone-on-bone OA, injections of HA or steroids are even less likely to be effective, and total joint replacement (TJR) may be a consideration. TJR surgery, performed about 800,000 times per year in the US for knee OA, can significantly reduce pain but has limitations. Even with complete removal of the arthritic joint surfaces, up to 20 percent of patients continue to experience pain after TJR.[8] These individuals are understandably perplexed. Their arthritic joint is gone. Why are they still hurting?

One of the reasons for persistent knee pain after TJR relates to the nerve supply for the joint. The nerves that supply sensation to the knee are sensitized by years of chronic pain. These nerves are further stretched and sometimes injured during the surgery. This can lead to continued chronic pain post-surgery. A procedure called a geniculate radiofrequency ablation is sometimes used to burn these nerves away from the joint. It can reduce chronic knee pain, but there are downsides. The ablative procedure isn't always effective. Even when it is, the nerves can regrow after a few months. With nerve regrowth comes a return of the pain. Fortunately, other potential options now exist, including nerve hydrodissections and regenerative therapies that I'll discuss in future chapters. Although I've performed many ablative procedures, I prefer, whenever possible, to restore nerves to health rather than destroy them.

Another reason someone may have persistent pain after knee TJR relates to the tendons and ligaments that have been strained and damaged over the years. Individuals with OA often have a gradual change in their joint angles as they lose cartilage. In the knee, a bow-legged appearance is typical (the medical term for this is a varus alignment). During TJR, surgeons typically correct this angle, reintroducing forces that the tendons haven't seen for years. The tendons and ligaments inside the "bow" are drawn tight, which can be painful given the rich nerve supply to those structures. Intensive post-surgical physical therapy helps most patients adapt to their newly restored angles, but sometimes, strain and pain can persist.

To understand the final reason for persistent pain after knee TJR, recall from Chapter 2, How to Damage Cartilage, that osteoarthritis pain is driven by the balance of cytokines in the synovial fluid, not the cartilage itself. TJR replaces the bone surfaces; the procedure does not replace the immune cells of the joint. If chronic inflammation persists within the capsule for any reason after TJR, so does the pain. It is possible to have a "perfect" joint replacement and still have pain.

Although joint replacement construction materials have become more durable over the past few decades, vigorous activity can still shorten the life of an artificial joint. Unlike your native joints, the body cannot repair or restore hardware. In this situation, wear and tear of the prosthesis does occur. About 50,000 revisions of knee replacements are done in the

US each year, a number expected to increase by 150 percent by 2040.[9] Worn-out hardware is often challenging to remove, and the new prosthesis may be less stable, frequently making revision surgery (and its recovery) more complex.[10] When I counsel patients considering TJR, I recommend that they do their best to be part of the "one and done" group. That means delaying or avoiding a joint replacement if you're an active fifty- or sixty-year-old.

For less advanced osteoarthritis (Grade 2–3) and related problems such as meniscus tears, arthroscopic knee surgery is common in the US and is performed over a million times yearly. Arthroscopy is a minimally invasive surgical procedure where small rigid tubes are inserted into the joint. One of the tubes is a camera (the arthroscope), and the others are instruments that cut, sew, or remove pieces of tissue. Inflammation that degrades cartilage in OA can also break down the meniscus, making it prone to tears. Although arthroscopy to "clean up" frayed or loose meniscus and cartilage in a knee with OA might sound logical, this surgery is no better than physical therapy and exercise in the long term.[11] I usually recommend that patients consider arthroscopic surgery if they are experiencing a "locking" sensation that prevents the full range of knee motion. In this situation, removing the obstructing piece of meniscus or cartilage can significantly improve their function. People who don't experience this locking sensation are usually better off spending time with a physical therapist, trainer, and walking partner than their surgeon.

Current treatments for osteoarthritis remain limited. NSAIDs have significant potential side effects. Repeated steroid injections accelerate cartilage damage. Hyaluronic acid injections frequently offer only minimal improvement. Arthroscopic surgery is no more effective than physical therapy. Even total joint replacement surgery fails to resolve pain in 20 percent of individuals. Novel approaches are needed for the problem of OA, moving beyond attempts to suppress inflammation and cover up symptoms. The focus should be on restoring the health of joint tissues with the therapies I'll discuss in later chapters.

Takeaways

1. NSAIDs can cause significant side effects when taken long term.
2. Repeated steroid injections can damage cartilage.
3. Joint replacement surgery should be avoided in younger, active individuals.
4. Arthroscopic surgery for osteoarthritis is no better than physical therapy.

Chapter 4

How Nerves (Mal)Function

Marcus was looking forward to an exciting year. His son was a starter on the high school football team, and his daughter was on her way to college. When not tossing a football around with his son or helping his daughter prepare for university life, he offered his do-it-yourself skills to the neighbors in his free time. Marcus could fix anything inside or outside the home. When neighbors needed advice, they called Marcus. On this particular Saturday, a neighbor called him to help clear an old stump from the backyard. Marcus gathered his shovel and a reciprocating saw. After digging around the stump, Marcus began sawing through the individual roots. The first root cut easily. The second one was thicker and deeper. He flexed forward to apply greater pressure on the saw and felt a lightning bolt of pain down his left leg.

When the pain hit, Marcus felt his leg buckle under, falling halfway into the small crater they had dug. He carefully lifted himself out of the hole, excused himself, and limped back to his house. He stopped at the medicine cabinet to find the anti-inflammatories and then headed to the couch to lie down. His leg was painful and slightly numb, and his back was in spasm. His wife returned home two hours later. Hearing the story and witnessing the groans whenever he tried to move, she helped Marcus into the car for a trip to the local urgent care. There, he received an

X-ray that showed some narrowing of the discs in his lower spine and was told by the doctor that he was experiencing sciatica. The term sciatica is used to describe pain in the sciatic nerve, which runs from the lower back to the feet. Sciatica describes where the pain is located but not its cause. Determining the cause often requires medical imaging, such as an MRI. The doctor ordered an MRI of Marcus's spine and prescribed oral steroids for his pain and muscle relaxants for his back spasms.

The oral steroids and muscle relaxants reduced his pain and spasms, and two days later, Marcus found himself lying on his back in the MRI scanner. He hadn't had an MRI before and was slightly startled by the thumping sounds and the claustrophobic feeling of being in a giant magnetic tube. He tolerated the experience, partly with the help of his muscle relaxants, and went home to wait for the results. His primary care physician called the next day, sharing that Marcus had a disc herniation causing severe compression of the spinal nerves.

Spinal discs are made up of fibrocartilage rings, like the meniscus of a knee. In the middle of the fibrocartilage rings is a gelatinous nucleus filled with proteoglycans. If you recall from Chapter 1, Joint Anatomy and the Myth of "Wear and Tear," proteoglycans attract and hold water, allowing the disc to provide a cushion between the spinal bones (the vertebrae). Also, like the meniscus, the fibrocartilage of a spinal disc can tear, allowing the gelatinous center to escape (herniate) and compress the nearby spinal nerves. Disc herniations can cause intense inflammation, pain, and sometimes numbness. When this occurs in the lower (lumbar) spine, it affects the spinal nerves that converge to form the sciatic nerve, sending pain all the way down the leg. This sciatica was what Marcus was experiencing.

A spine surgeon agreed to see Marcus the next day, recommending removal of the disc herniation to relieve the pressure on his spinal nerves. He told Marcus that without surgery there might be longer-term nerve damage. Marcus was taken to the operating room five days later. Afterward, the surgeon told him that the disc herniation was removed entirely and his spinal nerves were now free from pressure. Marcus felt rapid improvement in his leg numbness. Unfortunately, his back spasms continued, and he had sciatica pain whenever he was on his feet for more than a few minutes.

Marcus returned to work the following week with strict instructions from his surgeon to avoid all heavy lifting. He worked from his desk, frequently distracted by the back and leg pain. He began to see a physical therapist. The PT improved his strength, but his pain continued. Marcus's disc herniation was gone, and the surgery was a "success." Why was he still having shooting pain down his leg? Marcus wasn't alone. Most people will experience back pain at some point in their lives. And if they have spine surgery, there's about a 20 percent chance of chronic sciatica afterward.[1] To understand why persistent nerve pain like Marcus's occurs and what can be done to improve it, I first need to explain more about how nerves function in their healthy state. In the next part of this chapter, I explore this topic and the fascinating history of how the medical community grew to understand these specialized cells called neurons.

Nerve Functions: From Animal Spirits to Intricate Networks

It was around 170 CE that the Roman physician Galen first linked the action of nerves to the brain, not the heart. In his book, *On the Teachings of Hippocrates and Plato*, he conceptualized structures like hollow tubes that carried animal spirits to and from control centers in the head. In this theory, soft sensory nerves transmitted sensations, smells, and tastes, and hard motor nerves brought forceful spirits to power muscles. The concept of weightless, invisible *spiritus animalis* that controlled bodies remained the dominant paradigm of nerve function for over a thousand years.

This theory began to wane in the 1600s with writings on mind-body separation by philosopher-scientists such as René Descartes. While Descartes didn't dismiss the role of animal spirits, he increasingly attributed mechanical and physical properties to the function of nerves. Nonetheless, for another two hundred years, the model of nerves as simple tubes to carry messages persisted until the work of a brilliant Spanish neuroscientist, Santiago Ramón y Cajal. Ramón y Cajal used newly developed microscope techniques and an artistic hand to unfold the stunning complexity of the brain and peripheral nervous system (the nervous system outside the brain and spinal cord). Ramón y Cajal illustrated the intricate sprouting and branching of nerve cells (neurons) and the constant evolution of their structure and function. He studied the neuron's response to injury and made the first sketches of a cut nerve (Figure 4.1). In his sketches, the axon—the extended portion of a neuron that conducts impulses away from the cell's body—sprouts out, seeking to reconnect. He accurately depicted these cut nerves as a tangle of axons that today is called a neuroma—a benign mass of nerve tissue that often causes pain. Ramón y Cajal also drew gaps in the neural connections. These gaps are synapses that allow a signal to pass from one neuron to the next. This is where nerve signals are strengthened, weakened, and modified. He clarified that the nervous system was not a passive highway for brain traffic but a living, dynamic system continuously modified according to need and use. He gave us a visual depiction of how the brain

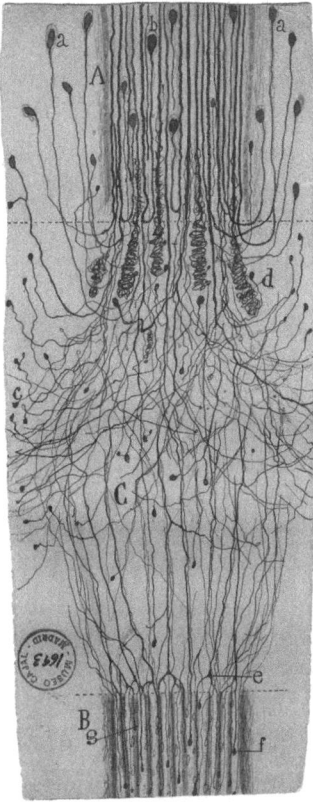

Figure 4.1. Illustration by Santiago Ramón y Cajal: The nerve "A" at the top of the image has been cut. It sends out a tangle of axons, ("C") that form a neuroma. Neuromas are often painful. https://commons.wikimedia.org/wiki/File:Santiago_Ramon_y_Cajal_cells_in_the_brain.jpg

and peripheral nerves "learn"—by strengthening the synapses between neurons and making new connections.

Ramón y Cajal won the Nobel Prize for Physiology or Medicine in 1906 for his insights and anatomic explanations for learning tasks. His work inspired generations of neuroscientists who followed. Teachers and coaches sometimes use the phrase "motor memory" to describe a person's ability to play a musical piece without the sheet music or hit the perfect basketball shot without thinking. These tasks, however, are better described as "neurologic memory," honed and strengthened by the neuron remodeling demonstrated in his illustrations.

Although Ramón y Cajal fully appreciated the anatomic intricacy of the nervous system, he did not yet possess the tools to understand the energy supplies needed to carry out learning and other essential neurologic functions. Neurons rely on a rich supply of adenosine triphosphate (ATP), a molecule that provides energy for all the active processes in living cells. ATP allows neurons to continuously pump sodium ions outside their cell membranes and maintain a strong electrical charge. When a neuron is activated, sodium channels open, and sodium ions flood in like a wave, rolling down the axon. Neuron firing and the wave of current that rolls down the axon is an all-or-none event. This means that the overall signal strength of a sensation or muscle action depends on how many individual neurons in a nerve are recruited and how frequently they fire. The signal travels through the peripheral nerves and across synapses to reach the spinal cord and, subsequently, the brain.

When a person practices a musical instrument or a jump shot, new synaptic connections are made, and synapses are reinforced along the path. If a person experiences chronic sciatica pain like Marcus, their body is also experiencing a type of learning. The neurologic signals from the pain of a disc herniation or surgery reinforce the connections with other pain and sensory systems. The longer the pain persists, the more the sensation is "learned." Removing a disc herniation may remove the stimulus but does not erase the synaptic connections made by the pain. The pain must be progressively trained away with physical therapy, exercise, and cognitive techniques.

Peripheral nerves contain sensory neurons, which carry information from the hands and feet to the spinal cord, and motor neurons, which transmit signals from the spinal cord to the muscles that control the hands and feet (Figure 4.2).

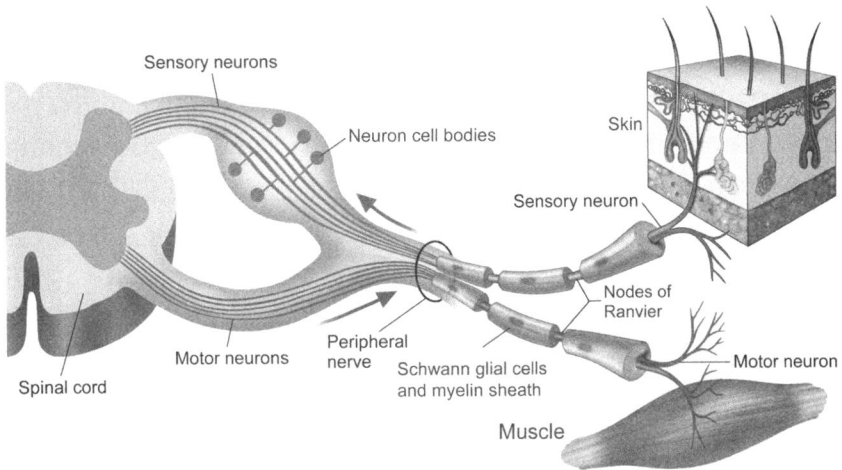

Figure 4.2. Nerve transmission: Peripheral nerves contain both sensory and motor neurons. These neurons are surrounded by Schwann cell myelin with intermittent nodes of Ranvier that significantly increase conduction speed. Neuron cell bodies are located near the spine, requiring long transportation distances for nutrition to the ends of the peripheral nerves.

These peripheral nerves can be quite long. The sciatic nerve, for instance, stretches up to three to four feet. Unfortunately, this length also makes the sciatic susceptible to damage and slow to recover. The neurons that make up the sciatic nerve manufacture many of the proteins and nutrients they require in the cell bodies, which are located near the spine. These nutrients must then be transported to the ends of the neurons in the feet. Therefore, when there is a disc herniation or other cause of sciatica, the neurons' energy and transport systems have to work overtime to repair the damage across long distances.

Support Structures for Nerves: Glial Cells

The advancements in microscopy techniques in the 1800s that allowed Ramón y Cajal to study the intricacies of neuron growth also aided the German scientist Rudolf Virchow in studying the billions of connective tissue cells between those neurons. Although these connective tissue cells had slightly different appearances depending on their locations, the cells consistently seemed to surround and stick to adjacent nerves. In his 1856 book *Cellular Pathology*, Virchow named these cells glia after the Greek word *kólla*, meaning glue. Virchow worked closely with Theodor Schwann, a German physician and physiologist. Schwann not only helped illuminate glia's structure and function but also coined the term "metabolism" and established cell theory, the concept that the cell is the basic unit of every living organism. The glial cells surrounding all the neurons in peripheral nerves are now named in his honor.

Schwann cells lie adjacent to neurons and produce layers of a protective, insulating sheath (myelin) that wraps around them like a blanket. The myelin wraps are not continuous. They leave regularly spaced gaps of exposed neurons (Figure 4.2 on page 43). These myelin gaps were first observed by French pathologist Louis-Antoine Ranvier, although he was not aware of their importance when he first observed them. Scientists now know that the "nodes of Ranvier" he discovered play a critical role in speeding up nerve conduction. When a nerve without myelin wrapping is activated, the signal rolls down the axon at a leisurely two miles per hour. If a nerve has a myelin wrap (with gaps), the conduction signal can jump from node to node at speeds up to 200 miles per hour, about the speed of a Formula 1 car. The Schwann cell myelin and its nodes of Ranvier allow humans to catch a falling object, hit the brakes of a car quickly enough to avoid a crash, and maintain balance on uneven surfaces. Without Schwann's glial cells, people would be slow, uncoordinated, and riddled with broken bones from constant falls.

The Squid and Its Giant Axon

My fascination with glial cells began in the late 1980s at the Marine Biological Laboratory in Woods Hole, Massachusetts. My research mentor, Dr. Michael Tytell, a neuroscientist at Wake Forest University, invited me to join him for a project at this historic Cape Cod laboratory. Scientists flock to this lab yearly to study marine creatures such as *Doryteuthis pealeii*, the longfin squid that migrates to the waters near Woods Hole each summer (Figure 4.3). The squid propels itself with lightning speed by jetting water through its hollow body, capturing prey, and avoiding predators. This rapid contraction relies on a specialized nerve, a giant axon that runs the length of its body. This axon is about 1,000 times the diameter of a human nerve and can be seen by the naked eye.

In the mid-twentieth century, scientists discovered the giant squid axon was large enough to accommodate experimental measuring probes and allow previously impossible neuroscience research on individual neurons. In the 1940s, Drs. Alan Hodgkin and Andrew Huxley inserted wire electrodes into the

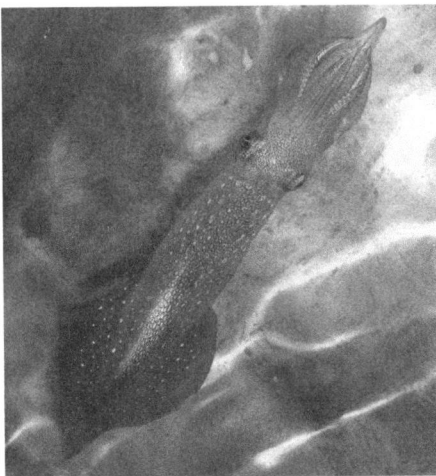

Figure 4.3. A live squid: The squid's giant axon runs along the length of the squid's body (approximately 14 inches in this specimen). (Image compliments of Michael Tytell, PhD.)

squid giant axon in their lab and detected the waves of electrical currents racing down the axon. Through their exacting work, Hodgkin and Huxley defined the fundamental physiology of nerve conduction and were awarded the 1963 Nobel Prize in Physiology or Medicine. Thanks to their work, those animal spirits described by Galen were now concretely measurable as sodium ions rushing in across the nerve membrane.

Doryteuthis pealeii also led me to the Marine Biological Laboratory in 1989 to study the interactions between its giant axon and surrounding glial cells. Using the same nerve dissection techniques described fifty years prior, my mentor and I bathed the squid's oversized nerve in fluorescent dyes. We then watched under a laser-light microscope as glowing packets of cell material streamed from Schwann cells to the axon.[2] These packets are vesicles, membrane-bound sacs, that carried protective proteins and molecules directly to the axon. The Schwann cells appeared to aid the axons at the time of injury. Thanks to the local Schwann cells, the axon did not have to rely solely on helpful molecules making the long journey from a distant cell body. They could also use their local first-aid stations—the Schwann cells. Thirty years later, it is now known that in addition to the vesicles I watched transfer in that Cape Cod laboratory, there are smaller ones, called exosomes, that the glia released. These exosomes, invisible to our microscopes at the time, deliver multiple protective factors that I'll discuss in future chapters.[3] Not only do glial cells speed nerve conduction, they also help support the axon at the time of injury.

Another type of glial cell, called microglia, is found throughout the spinal cord and brain. Microglia share the same lineage as the macrophages in joints and carry out similar immune-based functions. Like the macrophage at the time of injury, microglial cells also quickly release inflammatory cytokines such as IL-1 and TNF (see Figure 2.1, page 18). Microglia act at the cell bodies of neurons near the spine. When a nerve is compressed, stretched, or damaged, inflammatory factors from the microglia cause hyperactive firing and sensations such as electrical shooting and burning pain. Marcus's persistent sciatica after surgery indicated that he had microglial inflammation. Like the immune cell response in joints, this immune cell response to nerve injury causes pain but can also act to turn on repair mechanisms. I will discuss these mechanisms in greater depth in future chapters.

A Beautiful Battery: The Mitochondrion

The energy demands of a nerve are extraordinary. Nerves constantly pump sodium ions to maintain a charged electrical state, transport proteins down their axons, and shuttle vesicles and exosomes from surrounding glial cells. A rich supply of healthy mitochondria—structures in cells that generate energy in the form of adenosine triphosphate (ATP)—is critical. The high energy requirements of nerve action also explain why patients with neuropathy (nerve damage) from diabetes, chemotherapy, and metabolic diseases often experience symptoms first in their feet. Mitochondria must supply the energy needed to transport proteins and nutrients across the long distance of the sciatic nerve. This additional energy demand for long-distance transport—from the neuron cell bodies in the lower back to the feet—means that the feet are often the first to be affected in cases of metabolic or mitochondrial damage.

Most of the fuel for mitochondria comes from glucose (the simple carbohydrate and energy source found in all your cells) and fatty acids (an energy-rich long carbon molecule). Fatty acids are also the individual components of fats in the diet and the building blocks for many cell structures. These energy sources (glucose and fatty acids) are split up and shuttled as smaller fragments across the mitochondrial membrane. Splitting up glucose is a fast process and generates two molecules of ATP. Splitting glucose is one of the fuel sources your muscles would likely rely on if you're doing a forty-yard sprint or high-intensity exercise. If you're doing a lower-intensity exercise such as walking, your muscles have time to shuttle the glucose and fatty-acid split fragments into the mitochondria, where an extraordinary process occurs.

Once those glucose and fatty-acid fragments enter the mitochondrion, they generate high-energy electrons (e⁻, negative charge) and protons (H⁺, positive charge). The electrons power proteins called mitochondrial complexes that are critical for cell energy and life. If the mitochondrial complexes shut down for any reason (cyanide poison does this), it can be lethal. The positively charged protons are shuttled out of the center of the mitochondrion to a space between the inner and outer mitochondrial membranes (the intermembrane space). The shuttling of protons creates a batterylike gradient between the intermembrane space (high concentration of H⁺) and the inside of the mitochondria (low concentration of H⁺) (Figure 4.4). When the mitochondrion needs to make ATP, it opens a channel between these two spaces, the protons rush through, and ATP is generated. The brilliant efficiency of the mitochondrion makes 32 ATPs from a glucose molecule, 18 times more than the process of splitting the glucose apart.

The body processes fatty acids in a similar way as it processes glucose. Fatty acids are also split into short fragments and shuttled into the mitochondrion. Since fatty acids are long carbon chains, they create a greater number of fragments than glucose does. When a glucose molecule is completely run through the mitochondrion, it creates 32 ATPs. An average fatty acid yields

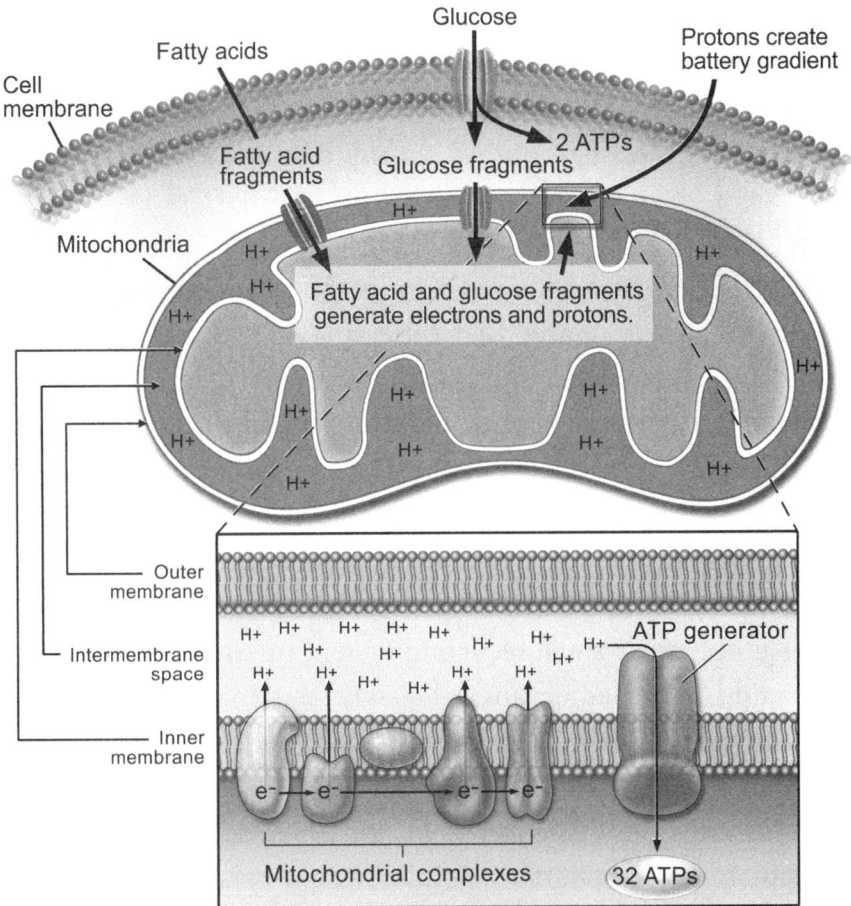

Figure 4.4. Mitochondrial function: Glucose and fatty acids are broken into smaller fragments. These fragments are shuttled into the mitochondrion to generate high-energy electrons (e^-) and protons (H^+). Electrons power the critically important mitochondrial complexes. Protons are shuttled to the intermembrane space, where they create a high concentration of positive (H^+) charges. When the mitochondrion opens a channel between the high H^+ concentration and low H^+ areas, protons rush through and drive the production of ATP that the cell uses for energy.

over 120 ATPs. For this reason, fatty acids that make up adipose (fat) tissues in the body are an efficient energy storage system. It is also notable that bodies efficiently use fatty acids during lower-intensity exercise—another reason to take that daily walk.

Cleanup and Repair Systems

The high-energy protons in the mitochondrion are needed to create the battery charge that generates ATP. But if the mitochondrion is damaged, and these charged particles are leaked, they can wreak havoc, damaging proteins and genes in the cell. Repairs must be carried out skillfully and efficiently. One of these repair mechanisms, autophagy, is critical to maintaining the cell's health and energy needs. The word "autophagy" comes from the Greek *auto*, meaning "self," and *phage*, meaning "to eat." Autophagy is a cell recycling system in all plants and animals and has helped organisms survive and evolve for the last 2 billion years. The vital cleanup process of autophagy employs tiny structures within the cell called lysosomes.

Lysosomes were discovered in the 1950s and were initially thought to be removers of cellular waste. With the advancement of microscope techniques in the 1960s, scientists became puzzled to find parts and even whole organelles (small functional structures in cells), such as mitochondria, inside the lysosomes. It turns out that this digesting organelle was more of a recycling center than a garbage dump. When a damaged mitochondrion meets the lysosome, mitochondrial autophagy recycles the mitochondrial parts, preventing the leakage of charged particles into the cell. Without autophagy, damage in cells, such as neurons, becomes significant. It comes as no surprise that defects in the autophagy process are linked to multiple neurological diseases such as Parkinson's, Lou Gehrig's disease (ALS), and peripheral neuropathy[4] (Figure 4.5).

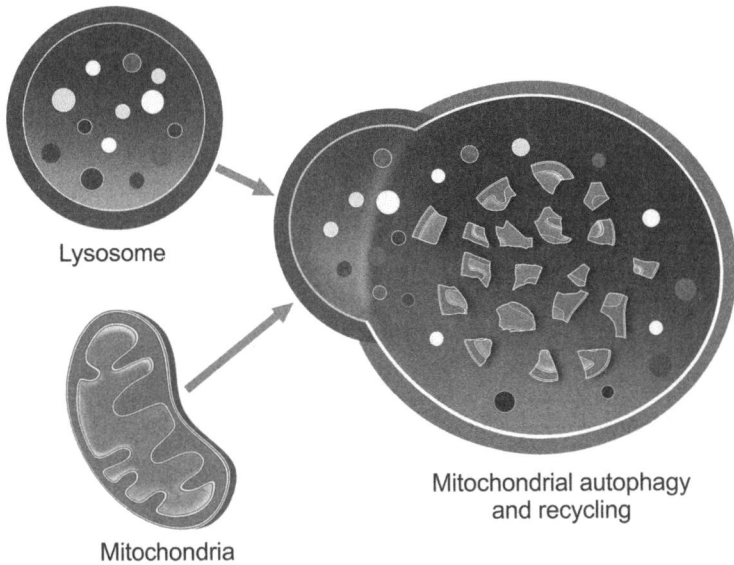

Figure 4.5. Mitochondrial autophagy: A damaged mitochondria fuses with a lysosome that digests and recycles the parts. This process prevents the release of damaging charged particles into the cell.

When Mitochondria Fail, Nerves Fail

Although neuropathy refers to dysfunction anywhere in the nervous system, this term is most often used to describe diffuse nerve disease following chemotherapy, diabetes, or viral infections. For example, paclitaxel, a chemotherapy used to treat breast, lung, and colon cancer, damages mitochondria and causes neuropathy in about half of the patients who take this treatment. Neurons examined with an electron microscope after paclitaxel exposure have swollen and deformed mitochondria. This damage impairs ATP production, slowing proteins and nutrient transport down the axon.[5] Long nerves, such as the sciatic nerve, are usually the first to be affected, causing numbness and tingling in the feet. Chemotherapy can also cause microglial cell activation, release of inflammatory cytokines, such as IL-1 and TNF, and significant nerve pain.[6]

Diabetes, with its elevations of blood glucose, is the most common cause of neuropathy in the US. With diabetes, nerve dysfunction is not only due to direct mitochondrial damage and microglial cell inflammation but also injury to the surrounding blood vessels. It's a triple hit for the nerves: Their energy supply is compromised, their blood supply is reduced, and they are chronically inflamed. About 50 percent of people with diabetes experience neuropathy at some point in their lives. About 20 million Americans are affected by these issues. Although neuropathies have many causes, mitochondrial dysfunction and chronic inflammation are common to nearly all.

Nerves are complex, energy-demanding structures that must continuously recycle and repair their mitochondria to maintain health and function. When damage occurs from a disc herniation, chemotherapy, or diabetes, patients frequently experience numbness and sometimes debilitating pain like Marcus. In the next chapter, I present the current methods to treat the pain of nerve injury and discuss why new therapies are needed.

Takeaways

1. Nerves are complex, highly regulated structures, not passive information highways.
2. Neuropathy pain is caused by the same inflammatory cytokines and proteins that drive osteoarthritis pain.
3. Mitochondrial damage and energy failure are common to most neuropathies.

Chapter 5

Current Nerve Treatments:
Relieve Pressure, Medicate, Inject

Marcus experienced a malfunction of his sciatic nerve from a disc herniation. The nerve compression was severe, causing numbness, weakness, and pain. His surgery was "successful," relieving pressure and restoring function, even though his pain persisted. After surgery, he tried several medications and received a steroid injection trying to resolve the residual pain. In this chapter, I'll discuss the pros and cons of the common therapies used to treat nerve compression and their effect on Marcus's sciatica.

Relieving Pressure at the Spine

Any compression of the lower spinal nerves can lead to sciatica. The two most common causes are disc herniations (like Marcus's) and spinal stenosis. A herniation results from a tear in the disc rings of cartilage in the spine and the sudden release of the disc nucleus material against the spinal nerves (Figure 5.1, page 54). If enough of the disc herniates outward and the compression is severe enough, it causes numbness and weakness. Fortunately, most disc herniations are smaller than Marcus's and do not require surgery. They cause inflammation of the nerves (and pain) but resolve with physical therapy and sometimes a medication or steroid injection.

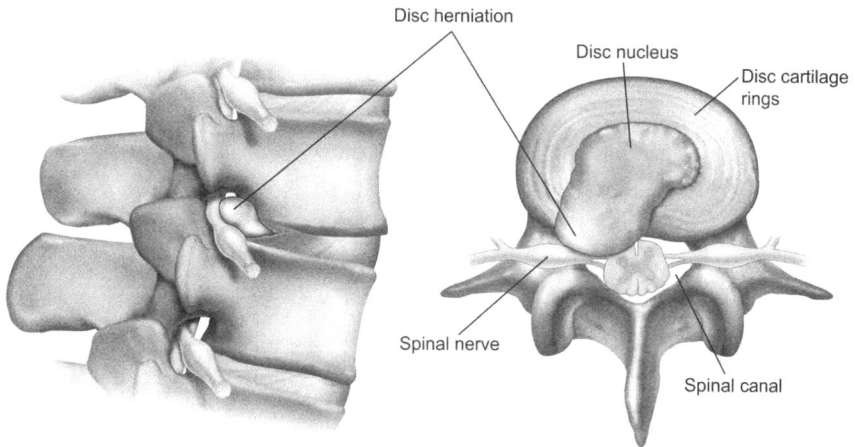

Figure 5.1. Disc herniation: With disc herniation, a tear in the disc rings allows the nucleus material to escape suddenly, compressing and inflaming the nearby spinal nerves.

Spinal stenosis is another cause of sciatica pain. Stenosis comes from the Greek word *stenos*, meaning narrow, and refers to the narrowing of the canal and the holes where the nerves exit. It results from osteoarthritis and the slow build-up of arthritic tissue, such as bone spurs (Figure 5.2). In the knee, bone spurs can be seen on X-rays around the joint and commonly cause stiffness (Figure 1.1, page 5). In the spine, these bone spurs not only cause stiffness but also encroach on the spinal nerves. As the arthritis worsens, the compression of nerves increases and can cause sciatica pain. Stenosis is a gradual process, and symptoms usually don't begin unless the compression is severe.

The decision to proceed with surgery is important and based on the degree of nerve compression. If the compression is significant enough to cause numbness and weakness, surgery will often help. If the individual is mainly experiencing pain (but

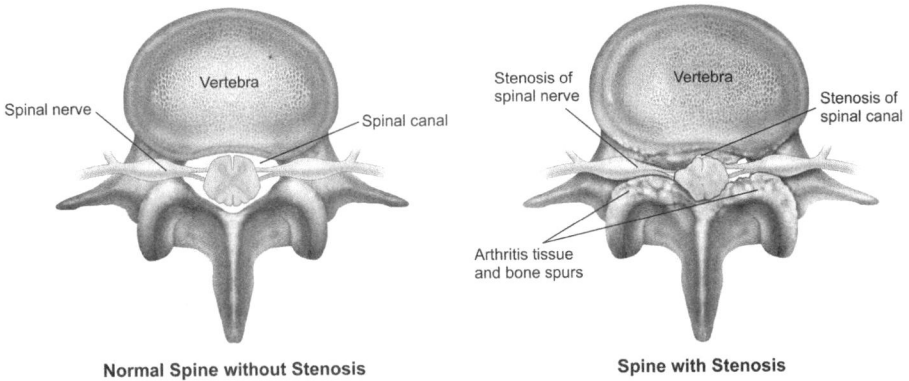

Figure 5.2. Normal spine and spinal stenosis: With stenosis, arthritis and bone spurs in the spine build up slowly, compressing the canal and the holes where the nerves exit. This can cause sciatica pain.

not numbness or weakness), conservative treatments (such as physical therapy) may be the best route. If you've ever had an MRI of the spine, there's a good chance that the radiologist has described some degree of stenosis or disc herniation. MRI images are now extraordinarily detailed—sometimes too detailed. They pick up every tiny piece of disc out of place and sometimes produce more questions (and anxieties) than answers. This level of MRI detail must be considered when deciding to proceed (or not) with surgery. A study published in *The New England Journal of Medicine* in 1994 (when MRI images were significantly less detailed) found that most individuals *without back pain* have spine abnormalities seen on MRI.[1] An MRI is a tool, but decisions for surgery should be based on a person's function and symptoms. Like knee osteoarthritis, spine pain isn't driven by what is visible in imaging studies. It's driven by inflammatory cytokines.

Relieving Pressure at the Peripheral Nerve

Like spinal nerves, peripheral nerves are also commonly compressed, especially at the wrist. Carpal tunnel syndrome (CTS) leads to over 600,000 surgeries per year in the US. CTS is caused by constriction of the median nerve as it courses through a tunnel in the wrist. The median nerve runs from the neck to the hand, providing critical sensation and the ability to move the hands and fingers with intricate precision. This tunnel, named after the adjacent wrist (carpal) bones, is narrow. If there is any swelling of the carpal tunnel, the median nerve becomes compressed, and the neurons that run to the fingers malfunction. The nerve compression causes the characteristic symptoms of CTS, including numbness, pain, and sometimes weakness in the hand. The median nerve dysfunction of CTS is similar to that seen in the sciatic nerve with a disc herniation or stenosis.

In contrast to the spinal nerves that make up the sciatic, the median nerve lies close to the skin surface and is easily viewed by ultrasound or tested with electrical nerve studies. Ultrasound can quickly assess the degree of nerve constriction and swelling. If the swelling is mild, patients often experience improvements in pain and numbness with physical therapy or injections. If the compression is severe, patients may do better with surgery to relieve the pressure and allow the nerve to recover.

It is also possible to evaluate the electrical function of the median nerve in CTS. Compressed neurons can lose their myelin coating, which can be electrically detected. Recall the discussion of Schwann cells from Chapter 4, How Nerves (Mal) Function, and the dramatic speed their myelin gives to nerve conduction. If this myelin coating is lost from compression, so is the nerve speed. If the pressure is relieved, the Schwann cells can regrow that myelin and restore nerve function—the numbness, pain, and weakness resolve.

For those suffering from spinal or peripheral nerve compression, physical therapy (PT) is also an invaluable method to relieve pressure on the nerve. PT has been shown to reduce pain and improve function with sciatica[2] and carpal tunnel syndrome.[3] A skilled physical therapist knows anatomy and body mechanics in depth. They can guide muscle, motion, and tissue work that improves symptoms for individuals suffering from nerve pain. If you have diffuse neuropathy (nerve pain that affects multiple body parts with symptoms such as numbness, tingling, and pain) from metabolic causes such as diabetes or chemotherapy, PT is also important. The PT techniques used for diffuse neuropathy will differ from those used to treat nerve compression. With diffuse neuropathy, the goals are to train balance and strength and reduce the risk of falls. Physical therapy and exercise can also improve nerve function with diffuse neuropathy, a topic I'll discuss more in future chapters. PT should be the first step for any spine or peripheral nerve disorder, optimizing function, decreasing nerve constriction, and reducing chances of injury.

Medicating to Suppress the Nerve

Coffee, breakfast, and an NSAID became part of Marcus's daily morning routine after his surgery. The NSAID didn't eliminate the sciatica pain. It just dulled it enough to get him through the day. But the pain was wearing him down. He spoke about it with his primary care physician, and she prescribed gabapentin (Neurontin) for his nerve pain. Marcus took the medication for a few weeks. He noted a decrease in his leg pain, but the gabapentin caused him to be so mentally cloudy that he couldn't function at work. He had to stop taking it.

Gabapentin was initially approved by the FDA in 1993 as an epilepsy drug. In initial studies, the medication's effect on the brain was not a side effect but a desired and necessary feature.

A few years later, research demonstrated that gabapentin also affected the peripheral nerves, decreasing irritability in neuropathy and associated electrical and burning sensations. In follow-up studies, gabapentin was found to improve the pain of both diabetic neuropathy[4] and shingles (post-herpetic neuralgia).[5] The positive results of these studies generated excitement for many neurologists and pain management specialists, who were frustrated with the limitations of other treatments.

I was doing my interventional pain management fellowship in the late 1990s, and many of the patients my colleagues and I treated had nerves that were malfunctioning from spinal compression, surgery, and injury. Gabapentin became one of the most prescribed medications. We knew of its cognitive side effects (especially at higher doses), but gabapentin's side effects were believed to be less risky than bleeding stomach ulcers from NSAIDs or overdoses from opioids. Gabapentin is still widely used. There are more than 60 million prescriptions for gabapentin written annually in the US.

Because of the mental cloudiness that Marcus experienced on gabapentin, his doctor switched him to pregabalin (Lyrica). This drug, which is similar to gabapentin, was approved by the FDA in 2004 for diabetic neuropathy and shingles. Unsurprisingly, Marcus found that the pregabalin also impaired his daytime focus. However, he tolerated pregabalin at night. It reduced his nerve pain and helped him find sleep.

I've spoken with many patients over the years who have had experiences similar to Marcus's with gabapentin or pregabalin. Those who rely heavily on cognitive processing during the day are sometimes the most sensitive to the side effects. Like an athlete who detects small changes in performance depending on training and diet, those who need their brains sharp are often the first to notice decrements in mental functioning.

Fortunately, many individuals tolerate gabapentin and pregabalin in the evening when the effects (and the side effect of sedation) are often welcome.

Because Marcus continued to experience ongoing sciatica pain despite his use of pregabalin and NSAIDs, his primary care physician asked me to see him for consultation. Marcus knew that I didn't prescribe opioids, which relieved him. He had watched a coworker struggle with opioid addiction and wanted to steer clear of that option. At our first meeting, Marcus and I talked about a couple of additional non-opioid options for nerve pain, including tricyclic antidepressants (TCAs) and serotonin and norepinephrine reuptake inhibitors (SNRIs). TCAs, including amitriptyline (Elavil) and nortriptyline (Pamelor), were developed as antidepressants in the 1950s. Although they are still used occasionally for the treatment of depression, this class of medications fell out of favor in the 1980s with the introduction of better-tolerated antidepressants, such as fluoxetine (Prozac). In low doses, TCAs have continued to play a role in the treatment of neuropathy pain.

TCAs affect neurotransmitter levels in the brain, spinal cord, and peripheral nerves. Neurotransmitters are found in the gaps between nerves and control the communication between those nerves. These chemicals explain how a nerve impulse can conduct across the synapses that Ramón y Cajal skillfully illustrated for us over a hundred years ago. Neurotransmitters such as norepinephrine and serotonin are not only involved in improving mood (why they are the targets of many antidepressants) but also in the reduction of pain. These neurotransmitters strengthen the synapses of pain-suppressor nerve pathways. TCAs can also cause sedation, dry mouth, urinary retention, worsening glaucoma, and cardiac arrhythmias. TCAs, especially amitriptyline, can also cause a drop in blood pressure when one stands up suddenly. While this side effect might be tolerated in younger individuals, it can put older patients at risk for falls, broken bones, and head injuries. Patients are usually told to take amitriptyline and nortriptyline in the evening when sedation may be welcomed for someone kept up at night with burning and shooting pain. Nighttime is also when people are most vulnerable to sudden drops in blood pressure, especially during a 3 A.M. trip to the bathroom.

Some studies have shown that the TCA amitriptyline may be more effective than gabapentin or pregabalin for neuropathy pain.[6] However, these study conclusions are based on doses often higher than many individuals tolerate. After discussion, Marcus and I decided that taking a TCA was not ideal for him, especially since his sleep had already improved on the pregabalin.

The next medication that Marcus and I discussed was duloxetine (Cymbalta). Like TCAs, duloxetine and related drugs such as venlafaxine (Effexor) are antidepressants that raise the concentrations of neurotransmitters such as serotonin and norepinephrine in the brain and spinal cord and strengthen pain-suppressor pathways. Duloxetine and venlafaxine produce less sedation and fewer side effects than TCAs. The effectiveness of duloxetine is similar to gabapentin and pregabalin.[7]

Since Marcus was seeking medication to treat his sciatica pain during the day, we decided that a trial of duloxetine was a good next step for him. Unfortunately, for the first couple of weeks, Marcus experienced nausea, a common side effect of these medications. Nausea occurs because of increased serotonin levels in the digestive tract and usually improves after a week or two. When I spoke with Marcus after a month, his nausea had resolved, and he noted that his pain was about 20 to 30 percent better. Duloxetine was certainly not a panacea, but it was helpful for him.

Freeing the Nerve with Injections

Often, individuals with chronic nerve or sciatica pain are stuck in a downward function spiral. Exercise causes pain, so they respond logically by doing less of whatever makes them hurt. This decrease in activity provides short-term relief but eventually results in additional weakness, poor body mechanics, and long-term worsening of pain. Physical therapy is critically important at this moment to regain strength and function, but many feel that they are unable to do exercises assigned to them by their PTs because of the pain. One of the potential tools that can provide an escape from the spiral is the epidural steroid or peripheral nerve injection.

With an epidural steroid injection, a needle is placed into the spinal canal near the area of compression caused by stenosis, disc herniation, or scar tissue. Corticosteroids, often accompanied by local anesthetics, are injected onto the painful nerves to reduce inflammation and pain. The first epidural steroid injection was performed in 1952, only two years after steroids were first applied to the knee to treat arthritis,[8] and their use has increased in frequency ever since. These injections of steroids into the spinal canal are now performed almost ten million times per year in the US. Their use is not without controversy. The most common criticism of these injections is their lack of long-term effectiveness.[9]

While I agree with detractors that steroid injections don't improve stenosis or change spinal anatomy, I believe the procedure can be effective when combined with physical therapy. A steroid injection can offer a patient a one- to two-month break from pain. This is often long enough for them to re-engage in a rehabilitation program and rebuild core strength. They're able to reverse the spiral and put themselves on a positive trajectory of strength →→ decreased pain →→ greater strength

→→ further reduced pain. The epidural steroid injection may not change their stenosis or disc herniation, but it can facilitate longer-term functional gains. A similar positive response can be seen with peripheral nerve injection in compressions such as carpal tunnel, where carefully placed steroids in combination with physical or occupational therapy can generate significant improvements. One caveat is that multiple epidural or peripheral nerve injections should be avoided whenever possible. Repeated steroid exposure can disrupt the normal immune processes that maintain the health of the tissues and nerves.

While spine injections have been traditionally performed with X-ray guidance, peripheral nerve injection procedures are increasingly performed with portable ultrasound. When physicians began using ultrasound in the early 2000s to guide peripheral nerve injections, we gained additional visual feedback on how the injected fluid (often corticosteroid mixed with a local anesthetic solution) affected the nerve. We could watch as the fluid mechanically separated the nerve from the surrounding tissues, creating a halo effect. The nerve injections were doing more than temporarily shutting down inflammation. They were also freeing the nerve from surrounding scar tissue or entrapment (Figure 5.3). This process of opening up the space around a nerve with fluid is called hydrodissection. Hydrodissection can be used to mobilize tissues and reduce nerve entrapment around spinal nerves as well as peripheral nerves. Combining injection and hydrodissection with physical therapy, can be an effective approach to reduce pain.

Marcus continued to have pain despite his medications and physical therapy, so we decided to get an MRI to look for residual nerve compression in his spine. In reviewing the images together, we could see the successful removal of the disc

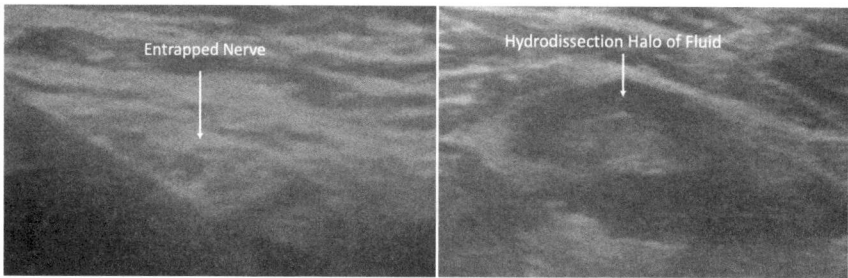

Figure 5.3. Nerve hydrodissection: Injections around nerves can be effective in hydrodissecting the nerves free from surrounding tissues and decreasing pain from scar or entrapment. (From the author's image files.)

herniation, but unfortunately, he had scar tissue in the area. This scar was wrapped around his nerve. The scar restricted the nerve as it exited the spinal canal and caused sciatica when Marcus exercised or stretched. We talked about treatment options. Surgery was not a good idea and could make the problem worse by adding more scar tissue. We also discussed doing an epidural steroid injection (with hydrodissection) of the nerve. Targeting the nerve as it exited the canal could free the nerve from the scar tissue. Marcus wanted to pursue this option and scheduled the procedure for the following week.

After obtaining X-ray views of Marcus's spine, I carefully placed a needle next to the problematic nerve as it exited his spinal canal. I injected a small amount of contrast dye to confirm the hydrodissection fluid would spread along the spinal nerve and his scar. I then started to slowly inject a diluted local anesthetic. Marcus, like most patients having this procedure, experienced a familiar electrical pain down his leg as the fluid traveled between the scar and his sensitized nerve. Although sometimes not pleasant, this sensation provides additional confirmation of the optimal placement of the fluid in the area of entrapment. Once the nerve was partially numb, I injected additional fluid to tease away the scar tissue and steroids to reduce inflammation and pain after the procedure.

Post-injection, Marcus had an expected flare-up of pain for a few days but then began noticing some improvement in his sciatica. He and I discussed that this was the optimal time for him to re-engage in physical therapy to mobilize the nerve and strengthen the surrounding muscles. Marcus's pain didn't completely resolve, so I tried repeating the epidural two months later. This second injection helped a little, but not as much as the first. At that point, we decided to hold off on any additional procedures and focus attention on his mobility and strength. Marcus has continued to make progress with his exercise program, which includes walking and strength training. He has returned to work, the gym, and the yard (but no more stump clearing).

Marcus responded to a combination of treatments. He had the spinal nerve pressure from his disc herniation relieved with surgery. He had sciatic nerve irritability and pain suppressed with medications. He then had scar tissue around his spinal nerves freed with hydrodissection during an epidural steroid injection. With these interventions and his exercise program, Marcus has continued to make progress. Nerves are specialized structures vulnerable to damage, and not everyone experiences similar improvements. Fortunately, for those who don't, there are ways to stimulate immune cells to augment natural healing. In the next chapter, I explore the foundation of healing and recovery: the immune system.

Takeaways

1. Surgery can help relieve severe compression of spinal and peripheral nerves.
2. Medications for neuropathy pain are limited in effectiveness and can cause side effects.
3. Injections can be helpful in hydrodissecting nerves from surrounding entrapment or scar tissue.

Chapter 6

Igniting the Immune System to Heal

Immune systems are powerful. They defend against bacteria, viruses, and even cancers. They also have the power to heal. In this chapter, I explain how white blood cells, proteins, and lipids strengthen joints and nerve function. I also discuss the similarities between chronic wounds and osteoarthritis and the critical differences between acute (short-term) and chronic (long-term) inflammation. In Chapter 3, Current Osteoarthritis Treatments, you learned how NSAIDs have multiple side effects and that repeated steroid injections may harm cartilage health. This chapter discusses the impact of these medications on the development of chronic pain and the immune-based mechanisms that restore health and improve pain.

Chronic (long-term) inflammation is universally harmful. The prolonged release of inflammatory cytokines and matrix enzymes damages joints and can lead to neuropathy and chronic pain. Because of the significant harm that occurs with chronic inflammation, many medical professionals have assumed that acute inflammation is equally toxic. Several scientific publications have expressed this concern, going so far as to say that acute (short-term) inflammation may even increase the chances of chronic pain. This fear of all inflammation (acute and chronic) has led to an explosion in the use of nonsteroidal anti-inflammatory drugs (NSAIDs). The message is that people must fight the immune response to injury with the same vigor that chronic autoimmune diseases such as rheumatoid arthritis or Crohn's disease are battled.

NSAIDs are recommended for aches, sprains, and strains and are part of standard protocols for treating acute pain after surgery. Despite assertions that NSAIDs are protective, research has never shown that NSAIDs reduce chronic pain if given at the time of injury or surgery.[1] The possibility that NSAIDs might actually *increase* the risks of chronic pain has not been considered. At least, not until now. To appreciate the disadvantages of constantly fighting acute inflammation, it is important to first understand the body's natural response to injury.

Immune Response to Injury

About ten years ago, I was playing a routine game of pick-up basketball with friends. Trying to work around a defender, I took an off-balance jump shot and landed with a twisting motion. This particular hard landing was a bit too much for my 45-year-old knee. I experienced immediate pain and swelling. An MRI confirmed my suspicion—a tear in my meniscus. Since my knee wasn't locking up and I could still work and ride an exercise bike, I decided against surgery. I dutifully took NSAIDs for a few weeks, combining them with my exercise program. The anti-inflammatory medication was quite effective in decreasing the immediate pain. My knee improved slowly, and after about six months, I mostly recovered. I avoided basketball but could bike, walk, and go for light jogs. When I look back now, I can't help but wonder: Did the NSAIDs slow my healing?

To understand the role of acute inflammation after an injury and the impact of NSAIDs, let's look at the body's response to a meniscus tear, ankle sprain, or any other injury you may have experienced. The first thing you'll probably notice is a bruise. The discoloration you see on the skin is from the injury to small blood vessels. These injured vessels activate platelets (colorless cell fragments in the blood that form clots), releasing hundreds of growth factors and proteins in the area. This "injury soup" ignites the immune system, which sends in its first responder white blood cell, the neutrophil. If the skin is broken, the neutrophil's job of removing bacteria and other invaders is essential to prevent infection. The arrival of the neutrophils releases multiple additional inflammatory cytokines and proteins. The result is inflammation, swelling, and pain at the site of the injury.

The neutrophils' proteins then attract a second wave of immune cells called monocytes. Monocytes travel in the blood and focus on the inflamed area, squeezing through gaps in the injured blood vessels. Once at the injury site, monocytes become agitated, growing and morphing into giant cells called macrophages, like Bruce Banner becoming the Incredible Hulk. These macrophages (which you learned about in Chapter 2, How to Damage Cartilage) quickly dominate the area. Macrophages secrete additional inflammatory cytokines and consume the first-responder neutrophils. If the immune system is working correctly, at this moment, a remarkable transition begins to occur. The macrophage stops its inflammatory rampage and morphs into an M2 cell. This M2 cell, like a subdued Hulk, starts to resolve the problem, producing growth factors, anabolic cytokines, enzyme inhibitors, and inflammation-resolving lipids (Figure 6.1, page 70). You will also recognize some of these players from Chapter 2. The M2 macrophage and the immune system become, in this way, resolvers of chronic inflammation and the foundation for healing and tissue repair.

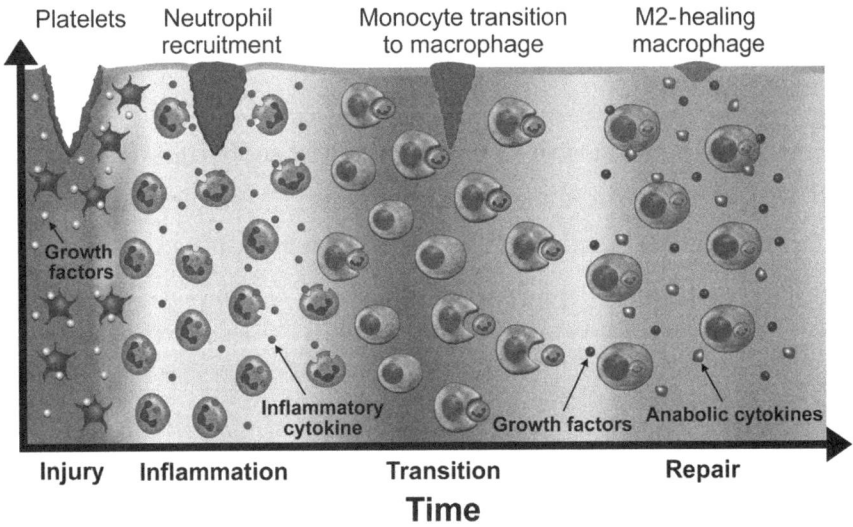

Figure 6.1. The healing cascade: Injury to tissues and blood vessels activates platelets and releases growth factors that attract white blood cells. Neutrophils arrive first to clean up the injury region. Monocytes then enter and morph into macrophages that consume neutrophils. If the healing cascade functions correctly, the macrophages then transition to M2 cells and release beneficial growth factors, tissue-building proteins, and inflammation-resolving lipids.

In the nervous system, a similar response to injury occurs. You may recall from Chapter 4, How Nerves (Mal)Function, that one of the glial cell types (microglia) shares multiple characteristics with macrophages. This is unsurprising as they originate from the same cell lines during development. When a nerve is injured, the body similarly unleashes a robust immune response. The microglial cell activates like a macrophage, producing inflammatory cytokines such as IL-1 and TNF. In a properly functioning immune system, microglia also transition to M2 cells. They become "resolvers," producing growth factors, anabolic cytokines, and inflammation-resolving lipids.[2] This beneficial immune cell transition struggles in the presence of diabetes and other metabolic disorders. The low-level, chronic inflammation of these diseases is enough to cause damage but not enough to engage the healing process. In these cases, re-igniting the immune system with exercise and the regenerative therapies discussed in future chapters is often necessary.

Osteoarthritis and Neuropathy Are Like Chronic Wounds

In Chapter 2, I presented the research on cytokine blockers and how they are ineffective for treating osteoarthritis (OA). The reason is that OA and neuropathy are more like chronic wounds than autoimmune diseases such as rheumatoid arthritis (RA). A nonhealing wound experiences a constant influx of white blood cells and their inflammatory products. The macrophages remain agitated and are unable to transition to M2 cells. IL-1 and TNF remain elevated. Tissue breakdown and pain are significant. Despite the chronic inflammation that is present in a nonhealing wound, a wound care specialist would not use a drug to suppress inflammation. Instead, they would look to methods to promote healing and tissue growth.

Like a nonhealing wound, OA and neuropathy represent a state of stalled healing in which inflammatory immune cells are continuously activated. The macrophage (in the joint) and the microglia (in the nerve) never transition to their M2 inflammation-resolving cells, and the diseases worsen. The concept of OA as a stalled immune cell transition is supported by research that analyzed the synovial fluid of individuals with knee OA. When the immune cells in the fluid were analyzed, researchers found that the ratio of activated macrophage to M2 cells correlated with the severity of OA on X-ray.[3] Where there were fewer M2 cells, the X-ray showed more severe damage. The cartilage and tissues were damaged because the immune cells never flipped the switch and became resolvers.

The similarities of OA and neuropathy to a nonhealing wound also explain a curious observation that physicians have noted for years in patients with painful tendons and ligaments. On ultrasound, chronically painful tendons such as the Achilles often "light up," displaying blood vessels that course throughout tendon fibers. This penetration of small arteries and veins deep into the tendon is not present in a healthy structure. The appearance of these new blood vessels is so prevalent that one of the treatments for a painful tendon is to mechanically scrape the blood vessels away. The rationale for this approach is straightforward. If an increase in blood vessels equals pain, then removal of blood vessels equals decreased pain. Instead of just removing them, doctors should also be asking *why* those vessels are there.

The body's natural response to an injury is to increase blood flow in order to deliver white blood cells, growth factors, and proteins for healing. After the body increases blood vessels and growth factors in the injured area, the next stage of wound repair is remodeling the tissues and restoring them to health. In this remodeling process, collagen fibers increase, fluid decreases, and blood vessels close down. When a painful tendon fills with excessive blood vessels, it is another sign that the natural repair process is stalled. It's an indication of a wound that hasn't healed. Although scraping away these blood vessels may help some patients, focusing on completing the healing process makes more sense. If the recovery process is completed, excessive blood flow (and the pain) in the area will also resolve.

NSAIDs May Lead to Chronic Pain

In 2022, Dr. Luda Diatchenko and colleagues at McGill University in Montreal, Canada, published a groundbreaking study that challenged existing dogma about the use of NSAIDs for acute pain.[4] The researchers asked a simple question: Why do half of patients with acute low back pain recover and the other half experience chronic symptoms? After analyzing multiple genetic and immune factors in these patients, they saw a clear pattern. Those who had a robust inflammatory response to their injury recovered. Those who had a weak immune response didn't. They knew this controversial result would be quickly challenged, so they repeated the analysis in patients with another condition—jaw pain from temporomandibular joint (TMJ) disorder. They saw the same result. Patients with a strong immune response were the ones who avoided chronic pain. Researchers then designed an experiment with mice that had inflammatory nerve pain. Without treatment, these mice resolve pain on their own after two or three weeks. If the researchers gave the mice NSAIDs or steroids, the treatments provided brief pain relief. (See Chapter 14, Autologous Conditioned Serum, for more information on these research techniques.) But the medications also blunted the immune response and actually *slowed* recovery. Just as it does with a chronic wound, an incomplete immune response to injury increases the risk of chronic pain.

Immune Stimulation May Reduce Chronic Pain

If immune suppression potentially increases the risk of chronic pain, does immune stimulation conversely reduce these risks? Drs. Chris Donnelly, Ru-Rong Ji, and their colleagues at Duke's Center for Translational Pain Medicine tested this question in the laboratory. They studied the effect of interferon proteins on pain. Interferons, which I introduced in Chapter 2, are released by the body in response to viral infection. You've probably experienced the effects of these potent immune stimulators if you've felt the fever, aches, and chills of the flu. Interferons can cause significant acute inflammatory pain. However, when Drs. Donnelly and Ji tested the interferon activities on *chronic* pain in laboratory animals, the effect was the opposite. Interferon and its acute immune stimulation worked to *resolve* chronic pain.[5]

Dr. Luda Diatchenko and the McGill researchers also found this link between immune stimulation and the resolution of pain. In their experiment where they increased the chances of chronic pain in mice by giving NSAIDs or steroids, if their research team injected neutrophils or neutrophil proteins into those same mice, they could re-establish pain relief. These immune cells (neutrophils) re-engaged the dampened immune system and reduced pain.

Additional evidence for the role of immune stimulation in reducing chronic pain comes from research collaborators Drs. Thomas Van de Ven and Chris Donnelly at Duke. Several years ago, Dr. Van de Ven and I studied the effects of nerve injury on pain in combat-injured soldiers. Many of these military service members had undergone additional surgeries, including leg amputation, because of their wounds. We followed the soldiers for months after their injuries, noting that about half of them resolved their pain. The other half, unfortunately, did not. We wanted to know why they had persistent nerve pain.

During their amputations, most of these soldiers also underwent a procedure called a traction neurectomy. In this procedure, the surgeon pulls tightly on the sciatic nerve before cutting it. The remaining nerve then retracts back into the muscle and away from the stump to prevent the nerve from being irritated by external pressure. This procedure reduces the chances of chronic pain, especially when the individual starts using a prosthesis to walk.

As part of our research, some of the soldiers agreed to let us keep and study their nerves that would have otherwise been thrown out. Over the past few years, Van de Ven and Donnelly have been analyzing these precious samples and the immune cells they contain. What they have discovered is an important step in understanding how nerves resolve pain after an injury. A greater concentration of neutrophils and macrophages at the nerve edge was associated with a *lower* incidence of chronic post-amputation pain.[6] Once again, a strong immune response appears to be linked to the resolution and improvement of pain.

Re-Establishing Balance

So far, I've presented evidence that a robust *acute* inflammatory response to injury is important to avoid (and treat) *chronic* inflammatory pain. To learn more, let's consider the four classes of molecules that acute inflammation and immune stimulation produce (Figure 6.2 on page 76). They are: anabolic cytokines, growth factors, enzyme inhibitors, and inflammation-resolving lipids.

In Chapter 2, you learned how cytokines, such as TNF and IL-1, are intensely inflammatory and can damage tissues if secreted for prolonged periods. You also learned how suppressing these inflammatory factors does not improve OA pain. For longer-term joint and nerve health, there must be a balance between the inflammatory and catabolic cytokines and the body's natural inflammation-resolving and anabolic cytokines. Several of these anabolic cytokines, such as IL-1Ra

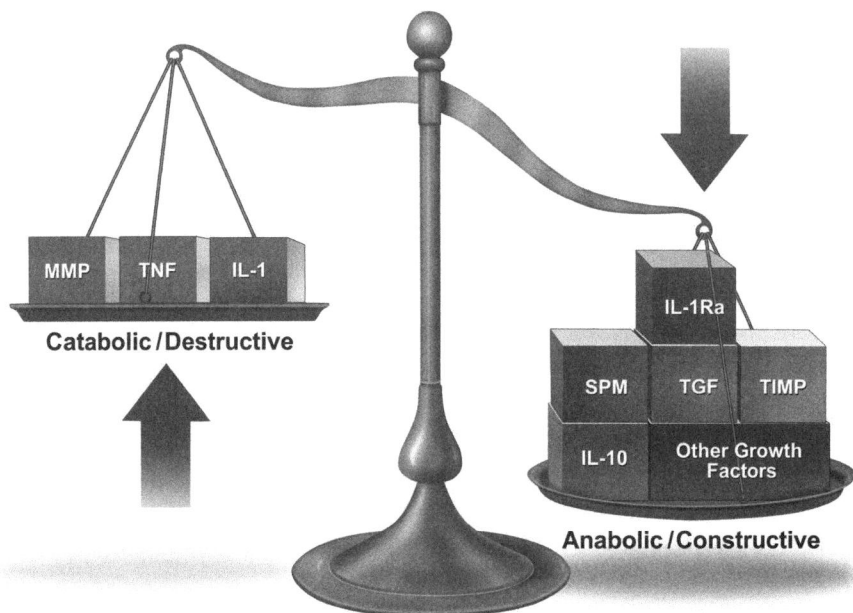

Figure 6.2. The balance of anabolic and catabolic forces: Joint and nerve health depend on anabolic (constructive) forces to balance (and outweigh) the catabolic (destructive) forces.

and IL-10, are quite powerful. Il-1Ra is a blocker that can naturally reduce the damaging effects and pain from the cytokine IL-1. IL-10 is produced during exercise recovery and is one of the reasons that exercise can reduce chronic pain. The production of these anabolic and inflammation-resolving cytokines by the M2 macrophage and microglia is critical to improving pain.

Another essential ingredient for tissue healing is growth factors. The body manufactures several hundred kinds of these small proteins. They help cells throughout the body grow and repair. Growth factors are often named according to function, such as nerve growth factor and vascular growth factor. One of these growth factors, transforming growth factor (TGF), is particularly crucial for cell recovery and pain relief. TGF is present in several of the regenerative therapies that I'll present in future chapters. Researchers have conducted various experiments to determine whether single growth factors can treat arthritic knees or injured nerves. These experiments often demonstrate that an individual growth factor can temporarily relieve pain but falls short of the complex tasks needed for complete healing. Growth factors work best as an orchestra rather than as solo instruments. Together, the concert of growth factors promotes the synthesis of proteins, collagen, and other components needed for healthy joints and nerves.

The third class of healing molecules produced with immune stimulation is enzyme inhibitors. Enzyme inhibitors are referred to as TIMPs (Tissue Inhibitors of MMPs). TIMPs are remarkably skilled at preventing damage from MMPs (matrix metalloproteinase enzymes) and other enzymes found in joints with OA. TIMPs help restore cartilage and prevent the breakdown of protective hyaluronic acid in our joints. Beyond inhibiting enzymes, TIMPs also play a role in reducing pain in neuropathy.

The fourth class of healing molecules is lipids. Lipids (which include fats and the inflammatory prostaglandins, introduced in Chapter 3) are sometimes maligned for promoting inflammation and disease. While this may occur with certain lipids, the criticism is not valid for the omega-3 fatty acids found in fish oil. We'll explore the health impact of various lipids in Chapter 7, Fats and Plant Colors to Resolve Inflammation. For now, I will just touch on omega-3s because of the products our bodies make from them. Omega-3 derivatives called specialized pro-resolving mediators (SPMs) can be tremendously effective in reducing pain. My collaborator, Dr. Ru-Rong Ji, has extensively studied the effect of SPM fatty acids on chronic painful conditions, especially after inflammation-associated nerve injury.

Pro-resolving mediators are released by M2 cells during the healing process and play a valuable role in stimulating the release of proteins and collagen to rebuild tissues. Several of these SPMs are called resolvins because of their ability to naturally resolve inflammation without disrupting the healing immune cascade. Other SPMs are called protectins. Protectins function to protect nerves and reverse damage at times of injury or stress. These omega-3 fatty acid derivatives are critical to reduce osteoarthritis and neuropathy pain.

These four healing mechanisms (anabolic cytokines, growth factors, enzyme inhibitors, and inflammation-resolving lipids) work together to restore balance, improve tissue health, and reduce pain.

I recently had my own (unfortunate) opportunity to re-test the relationship between injury, acute inflammation, and healing. Running on a trail in the woods and making a left turn, I failed to see a large rock obscured by a pile of leaves. My left foot held tight, but the rest of my body continued forward and sideways. I tried to recover with my right leg but ultimately found myself in a twisted mess on the trail. I slowly stood up, humbled and bleeding, and hobbled home. Sadly, that hobbling continued. An MRI confirmed that I had suffered a second meniscus tear in my knee and a partial tear in my medial collateral ligament (inside of my knee). It was more painful than the tear I had experienced ten years prior, probably due to the additional ligament damage. I spoke with an orthopedic colleague who agreed that surgery wasn't needed. I am well into my fifties, my knee wasn't locking up, and my medial collateral ligament wasn't completely torn. She gave me the standard advice and recommendations—anti-inflammatories and physical therapy—and advised me to consider a steroid injection if the pain became too severe.

This time, I decided on a different recovery path. I avoided taking any NSAIDs and declined a steroid injection. The pain was rather impressive. I limped around for a couple of weeks and endured sarcastic comments from colleagues who questioned my sanity for foregoing the accepted treatments. After a few days, I could ride an exercise bike again at a gentle pace, although my muscles quickly weakened. I had a deadline: a family ski trip scheduled in less than a month that I didn't want to miss. Timing for injuries is never ideal. I continued my strength work and rehab guided by an excellent physical therapist. After about three weeks, the swelling began to subside, and I felt a "switch flip" with my knee. The pain improved and my strength increased.

I made the ski trip. I didn't quite keep up with the adventurous teenagers in our group and their desire to continuously ski in the trees, but my runs were solid and injury-free. More importantly, the time with family and lifelong friends was tremendously heartwarming. Even though the damage to my knee was more significant in the second injury, my functional recovery was considerably faster. My immune system pumped out anabolic cytokines, growth factors, enzyme inhibitors, and inflammation-resolving lipids without the hindrance of anti-inflammatories, which I believe sped my recovery.

Our body's immune response to injury is a potent tool to reduce chronic pain. Yet the dogma of "fighting acute inflammation" is entrenched in the medical system and on pharmacy shelves. Thankfully, a paradigm shift toward therapies that enhance rather than suppress immune function is occurring. To accomplish these healing activities, immune cells also require raw materials to produce the growth factors, cytokines, and lipids that allow the body to resolve inflammation. Those vital building blocks are found in food and are the topic of the next chapter.

Takeaways

1. Acute inflammation can "flip" the immune switch and produce inflammation-resolving macrophages that heal tissues and reduce chronic pain.
2. Laboratory studies show that medications that shut down acute inflammation may increase the risks of chronic pain.
3. Treating chronic pain requires the orchestration of multiple immune-based healing factors.

Chapter 7

Fats and Plant Colors
to Resolve Inflammation

The body's immune cell activities play a critical role in determining whether people experience chronic inflammation and pain or can "flip the switch" to begin resolving that inflammation. Crucial components of this immune-based healing responses are the omega-3 derivatives called specialized pro-resolving mediators (SPMs). SPMs, such as resolvins and protectins (introduced in Chapter 6, Igniting the Immune System to Heal), are produced by M2 macrophage cells from the healthy fats in the diet. SPMs, in combination with plant color compounds, are powerful tools to reduce pain.

Resolving, Not Fighting, Inflammation

"Resolving" and "fighting" inflammation may sound like similar concepts, but there are important differences. Patients typically fight inflammation by shutting down inflammatory pathways with medications such as nonsteroidal anti-inflammatory drugs (NSAIDs), corticosteroids, and rheumatoid arthritis (RA) drugs. NSAIDs turn off the enzymes that produce inflammatory prostaglandins. Steroids suppress inflammatory immune cell function. RA drugs shut down inflammatory cytokines. Fighting inflammation can be effective in temporarily reducing pain. But this immune suppression (as I discussed in Chapter 2, How to Damage Cartilage, and Chapter 3, Current Osteoarthritis Treatments) doesn't slow or reverse osteoarthritis (OA) or neuropathy. The medications that fight inflammation can also produce significant side effects if taken long-term.

On the contrary, resolving inflammation is a natural process that engages the immune cells in a healing cascade discussed in Chapter 6. If an immune stimulus (such as acute inflammation or exercise) activates the M2 macrophage to produce growth factors, inflammation-resolving cytokines and SPMs, the body starts to repair joint cartilage, rebuild mitochondria, and restore nerve function.

Fats, Fatty Acids, and Their Shapes

So far, in this chapter and this book in general, I've talked about "fats" but not "oils." I do this to avoid confusion about these substances. The distinction between "fat" and "oil" is generally based on what the substance looks like at room temperature. If it remains a solid (like butter or lard), it is typically called a fat. If it is a liquid, people usually call it an oil. But what if the temperature of your room changes? If butter left on the counter in the summer melts, has it become an oil? If olive oil is put into the refrigerator and congeals, is it a fat? Rather than be preoccupied with temperatures, it's less confusing to call them fats, especially since all fats and oils are composed of mixtures of fatty acid building blocks. I'll continue to use the term "fats" to describe the fats and oils that people use in the kitchen, except when I want to mention an oil specifically, such as olive oil, or corn oil.

Recall from Chapter 4, How Nerves (Mal)Function, that fatty acid chains are broken down and shuttled into the mitochondria to generate ATP. Fatty acids are a critical source of fuel for cells. In addition to their role in energy storage, fatty acids regulate multiple immune functions, including inflammation. The immune system impact of fatty acid chains is partially driven by their shape: straight, curved, or bent (Figure 7.1).

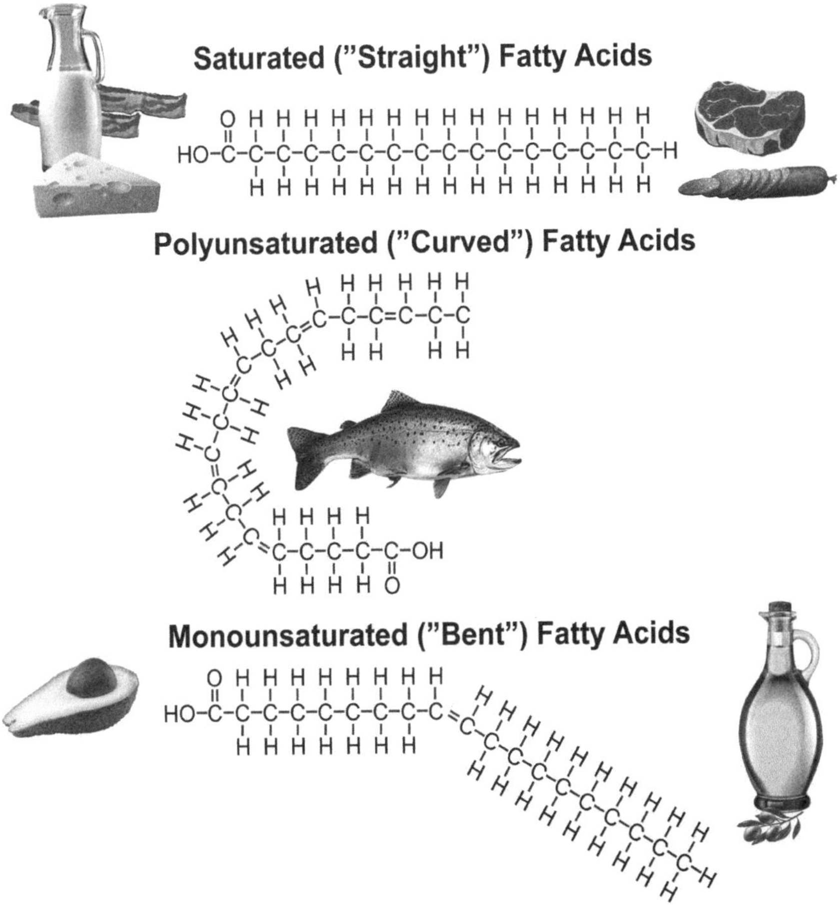

Figure 7.1. Types of fatty acids: Saturated (straight) fatty acids are found in red meats, cheese, and milk. Polyunsaturated (curved) fatty acids are found in fish. Monounsaturated (bent) fatty acids are found in olive and avocado oil.

Saturated (Straight) Fatty Acids

Saturated fatty acids are straight. The long carbon chains have rows of hydrogen atoms on each side and no room for anything else. They are "saturated" with hydrogen. The unbroken rows of hydrogens allow these fatty acids to pack together tightly so they form solids at room temperature. The stable structure of saturated fatty acids makes them less prone to spoiling over time.

The shape of saturated fatty acids also dictates how they affect cells. Each cell of the body is surrounded by a membrane that holds and protects the cell's contents. These cell membranes are made of approximately 50 percent fatty acids, constructed from the fats that people eat. Once the body consumes them, it breaks down fats into fatty acids and transports them in the bloodstream to targets throughout the body. Fat is delivered to the cell membranes of nerves, joint tissues, and even the blood vessels themselves. When incorporated into the membranes of cells, saturated fatty acids provide structure. However, a diet too rich in these straight fatty acids can result in excess rigidity in cell membranes. Stiffness is particularly problematic with structures such as arteries that must expand and contract with each beat of the heart. Consuming larger quantities of food that are rich in saturated fatty acids, such as lard, meats, and cheeses, can stiffen cell membranes and potentially contribute to vascular diseases such as high blood pressure.

In addition to their physical effects on the cell membranes, saturated fats can also alter immune function, causing macrophages to produce inflammatory cytokines such as IL-1. These inflexible fatty acids activate macrophages without letting them transition to M2 cells. Inflammation, therefore, does not resolve, and the macrophages continue their prolonged release of IL-1, damaging the cells around them and their mitochondria. Mitochondrial injury is particularly problematic for energy-hungry neurons that are constantly transporting nerve signals and nutrients along their long axons (see Chapter 4 and 5.)

In laboratory studies, saturated fats slow transportation activities and contribute to neuropathy, especially if diabetes is also present.[1] Excessive consumption of saturated fats can have harmful consequences not only for blood vessels but also for nerves.

Polyunsaturated (Curved) Fatty Acids

Polyunsaturated fatty acids have multiple areas where their carbon chains aren't saturated with hydrogen atoms (see Figure 7.1). These unsaturated areas in a fatty acid produce multiple kinks in the molecule and a resulting curved structure. Polyunsaturated fatty acids don't line up well and usually remain liquids, even in the refrigerator. The location of the kinks in the structure is also critical for fatty acid function. If the first kink is near the front of the fatty acid chain, the fatty acid is called an omega-3, providing benefits that I'll present in a moment. If the first kink is later in the chain, the fatty acid is called an omega-6.

The content that follows includes details about the different kinds of polyunsaturated fatty acids.

Omega-6s. Omega-6 fatty acids are found in many vegetable (and seed) oils such as corn, soybean, and canola. The body can't manufacture these fatty acids, making it essential that people consume omega-6 fatty acids in their diets. Although some consumption is necessary, global consumption of these fatty acids has ballooned with the industrialization of food in the last century. The challenge with this rise in omega-6 consumption is how the body metabolizes them. In addition to being used as fuel for mitochondria, omega-6s are converted to prostaglandins. Recall from Chapter 3, that prostaglandins are the inflammatory molecules that patients often take NSAIDs to suppress. A multicenter study published in the journal *Osteoarthritis and Cartilage* examined the impact of omega-6s on inflammation in approximately five hundred individuals with knee OA. When researchers analyzed the fatty acids in the blood and inflammation on knee MRIs, they found a clear correlation.[2] The greater the omega-6s, the more the joint inflammation. Laboratory research has also shown that diets high in omega-6 can slow mitochondrial function, damage neurons, and increase pain.[3] If a person's consumption of omega-6 fatty acids exceeds what the body needs, it can contribute to chronic inflammation and pain.

Trans-fatty Acids. The multiple kinks in polyunsaturated fatty acids not only make them curl but also cause them to be unstable and spoil more quickly than saturated fats. This instability presented problems for food manufacturers trying to ship products across the country. It was discovered that hydrogen atoms could be added to liquid vegetable oils, turning them into more solid (and stable) saturated fats such as margarine and shortening. This process of "hydrogenation" was quickly adopted, significantly increasing the shelf lives of many manufactured foods.

But there was a side effect to this hydrogenation process. When vegetable oils were treated with hydrogen, about a third of the kinks in the fatty acids didn't saturate with hydrogens. Instead, they just flipped directions. The Latin term for this change in direction is *trans*. The process of making vegetable oils more shelf-stable created trans fats that were even more inflammatory than saturated or omega-6 fats. Over the past few decades, the potential harms from trans-fatty acids have been repeatedly shown in research studies. The FDA now bans trans fats in concentrations beyond 0.5 grams/serving.

That means that trans fats aren't completely gone, but they are reduced.

Omega-3s. If the first kink in a polyunsaturated fatty acid is near the beginning of the carbon chain, it forms an omega-3. Omega-3s are highly concentrated in cold-water fish such as salmon, anchovies, sardines, and tuna, and are often called "fish oils." The specific types of omega-3 fish oils that provide benefits for joints and nerves (and hearts) are EPA and DHA. These acronyms stand for long chemical names that many scientists often don't remember and that I will leave out here. You may have seen EPA and DHA on labels if you've looked at fish oil supplements. Other kinds of omega-3s are also abundant in plant sources such as flaxseed, walnuts, and other nuts. Plant-based omega-3s differ from those found in fish. An additional step is required for the body to convert these plant-based versions into active EPA and DHA (Figure 7.2, page 89). Only about 5 to 10 percent of plant omega-3s convert. So a higher dose is required if you're supplementing with a plant rather than a fish source. EPA and DHA can resolve inflammation, and supplements of these omega-3s have been shown to reduce pain and improve joint function in individuals with OA.[4] Higher omega-3 consumption is also associated with healthier cartilage on MRIs of the knee.[5]

The role of omega-3s for nerve health has also been studied. Recall that mice fed high concentrations of omega-6 fatty acids will develop nerve pain. If those same mice switch their diet and increase the concentrations of EPA and DHA, their nerve pain resolves.[6] These benefits have also been seen in human patients. DHA/EPA supplements have been shown to reduce the incidence of peripheral neuropathy in women receiving chemotherapy for breast cancer.[7]

The potential reductions in pain with omega-3s prompted researchers at the University of North Carolina and the National Institutes of Health to test the effect of these polyunsaturated fats on patients experiencing persistent and severe headaches. The investigators randomly assigned individuals to receive either a typical diet, a diet supplemented with omega-3-rich fish, or a diet supplemented with omega-3-rich fish with a simultaneous reduction in omega-6 vegetable oils.[8] After four months, researchers measured blood levels of inflammation-resolving SPMs and re-assessed headache frequency. Both of the groups that received omega-3 supplements had increased levels of SPMs and decreased headache frequency. The groups that *increased* omega-3s and *decreased* omega-6s experienced the most significant reductions in headaches. Changing the ratio of fats in their diet decreased their pain.

One way that EPA and DHA benefit the body is through immune cells such as the macrophage. The macrophage converts EPA and DHA to SPMs, such as resolvins and protectins. EPA and DHA not only supply the raw materials to make SPMs, but they also assist the macrophage in transitioning to an M2 cell to manufacture these inflammation resolvers. EPA and DHA are critical ingredients for immune systems to resolve inflammation, reduce pain, and restore nerve function after injury (see Figure 7.2).

Monounsaturated (Bent) Fatty Acids

Monounsaturated fatty acids such as those found in olive and avocado oil have only one kink in their structure. Their single kink bends the fatty acids and prevents them from lining up tightly like saturated fats do. This means monounsaturated fatty acids are usually liquid at room temperature. However, if the room gets cold (or you put them in the refrigerator), they

Omega-3 Polyunsaturated Fatty Acids

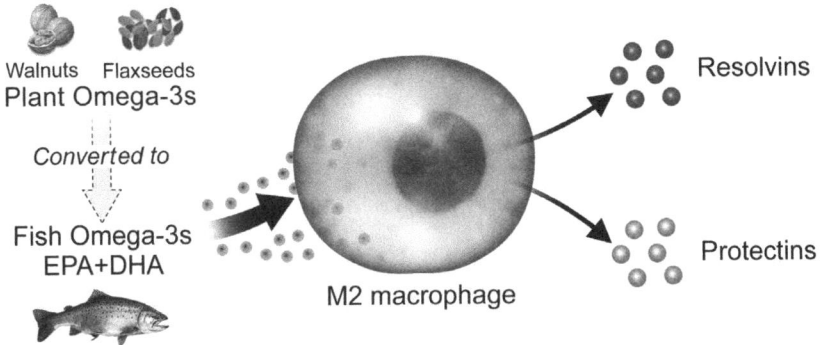

Walnuts Flaxseeds
Plant Omega-3s

Converted to

Fish Omega-3s
EPA+DHA

M2 macrophage

Resolvins

Protectins

Figure 7.2. Omega-3 fatty acids: Omega-3s, such as fish-derived EPA and DHA, are used by the M2 macrophage to produce resolvins and protectins that resolve inflammation. Plant sources of omega-3s (such as flaxseed and walnuts) must first be converted in the body to active forms of EPA and DHA. Only 5 to 10 percent of plant omega-3s make the conversion.

will solidify. Like omega-3s, olive oil helps macrophages transition to M2 cells and begin the process of resolving inflammation and rebuilding tissues.[9] Olive oil also reverses some of the mitochondrial damage produced by saturated and omega-6 fatty acids.[10] That makes this bent fatty acid good for nerves as well as joints.

The effects of olive oil (monounsaturated fatty acids) and nuts (polyunsaturated omega-3s) were tested for Spanish individuals with diabetes or other cardiac risk factors. In a multicenter study published in *The New England Journal of Medicine*, investigators randomly assigned participants to either a low-fat diet, a regular diet with an olive oil supplement, or a regular diet with an omega-3 nut supplement such as walnuts. After 4½ years, the reductions in heart disease in the groups that received olive oil or nut supplements were so significant that the researchers stopped the study early.[11] It would have been unethical to allow individuals to continue with a diet without one of these supplements. The benefits of olive oil and nuts in this study were undeniable. But the fatty acids weren't the only components of these food supplements that improved health. Olive oil and nuts also contain compounds called "flavonoids."

Plant Colors for Joint and Nerve Health

You may have heard the phrases "eat the rainbow" and "eat more colors." The reason behind this dietary advice is a family of plant compounds called "flavonoids." Flavonoids give plants their flavor, their deep red, blue, purple, orange, and green hues, and their health benefits. Berries are rich in flavonoids. So are other fruits, vegetables, green teas, and dark chocolate. Flavonoids have been studied for years, and several have been developed into commercial supplements. You may have heard of some of these flavonoids, such as "quercetin" (found in apples, kale, onions, and green tea), "resveratrol" (found in red grapes, blueberries, and blackberries), and "curcumin" (found in turmeric). While individual flavonoids offered in commercial supplements may offer health benefits, it's important to remember that the fruit or vegetable that makes these compounds also produces hundreds of others like it. You can take a supplement. You can also enjoy the rich foods that provide a rainbow of flavonoids.

One of the reasons that plants make flavonoids is to protect themselves. A fruit or vegetable grown under the threat of heat, cold, fungus, and insects has greater concentrations of flavonoids than one raised in a protected environment. This is the reason that fruits and vegetables grown in our backyards or sold at the farmers' market are likely better for us than their greenhouse cousins. Flavonoids that protect the plant also protect us.

One of the ways flavonoids provide this protection is by cleaning up inside the cell and resolving inflammation. Recall from Chapter 4, that mitochondria produce highly charged particles to power their ATP energy machinery. When mitochondria malfunction, these charged particles escape, damaging proteins, DNA, and other vital cell components. Flavonoids act as "scavengers," clearing and removing these damaging particles and the chronic inflammation they produce. Flavonoids such as curcumin (found in turmeric) also decrease inflammatory cytokines such as IL-1 and TNF, and enzymes such as MMP. Flavonoids further enhance M2 macrophage production of SPMs, such as resolvins and protectins.[12] This combination of flavonoid effects improves cell functions, reduces chronic inflammation, and re-establishes the balance of cytokines and growth factors needed for joint and nerve health.

The Power of Combining Healthy Fats and Plant Colors

Multiple studies have confirmed the benefits of eating a diet that combines omega-3s (fish and nuts), monounsaturated fats (olive oil), and flavonoids (colorful fruits and vegetables). This research began with the observations in the 1950s that multiple societies around the Mediterranean Sea experienced less heart disease. Although no uniform diet exists in these populations, individuals in these Mediterranean countries commonly consume greater quantities of fish, nuts, olive oil, fruits, and vegetables. Diets rich in these ingredients have been shown to not only reduce heart disease but also protect cartilage. In 2018, researchers from Padova, Italy, found a correlation between a Mediterranean diet and knee cartilage thickness. They studied 780 individuals who had MRIs of their knee osteoarthritis. The investigators found that those who consumed more fish, olive oil, fruits, and vegetables had thicker cartilage. These foods protect joints from developing OA.[13]

The nutrients in fish, olive oil, fruits, and vegetables don't "fight" inflammation—they resolve it. These foods provide the raw materials to "flip" the immune switch and produce the resolvins, protectins, growth factors, and inflammation-resolving cytokines that joints and nerves need for long-term health. Combining these foods with exercise, which I'll discuss in the next chapter, generates a tremendously powerful stimulus for healing.

Takeaways

1. The industrialization of food over the past century has changed the kinds of fats people consume and likely worsens chronic inflammation and pain.

2. Omega-3s are used by M2 macrophages to produce resolvins and protectins that resolve inflammation and reduce pain.

3. Plant colors (flavonoids) protect cells, reduce chronic inflammation, and complement the benefits of omega-3s, olive oils, and nuts found in a Mediterranean diet.

Chapter 8

Exercise, Inflammation, and Joint Healing

When Sarah went to her doctor for her osteoarthritis pain, the first prescription she received (along with her NSAID) was for physical therapy. Physical therapy, while perhaps less headline-catching than the latest procedure, was one of the most important things Sarah could do for the health of her joints. Exercise increases the strength of muscles, tendons, and ligaments and improves cartilage health. Exercise also reduces osteoarthritis pain. The risks of exercise are low, and the cost is even lower. Exercise provides these benefits by *causing* acute inflammation and turning on the body's repair mechanisms.

Inflammation and Tissue Repair

Working out—whether a brisk walk, a jog, or a pickleball game—stresses muscles, tendons, ligaments, and cartilage. Higher-intensity exercise may even cause tiny tears (microinjury) in these tissues. These stresses and microinjuries activate white blood cells, such as the macrophage, and release inflammatory cytokines, such as IL-1 and TNF (which you learned about in Chapter 2, How to Damage Cartilage).[1] With exercise, an additional inflammatory cytokine, IL-6, is released in large concentrations. IL-6 has a wide range of effects and is particularly important to turn on post-exercise muscle repair and strengthening mechanisms.[2]

The acute inflammation from exercise acts as an immune stimulant. This stimulation causes the macrophage to transition to an M2 cell. It then begins producing the anabolic cytokines (such as IL-1Ra and IL-10), growth factors (such as TGF), and inflammation-resolving lipids (such as resolvins and protectins) that you read about in Chapter 6, Igniting the Immune System to Heal, and Chapter 7, Fats and Plant Colors to Resolve Inflammation. These factors work together to strengthen tendons and muscles and increase the production of collagen and proteoglycans in cartilage.[3] In this way, the acute inflammation of exercise leads to long-term benefits.

Being mildly sore for a couple of days after a workout is okay and common. It is a sign that you have stressed your muscles and joints and have likely turned on many of your body's tissue-building mechanisms. That said, exercise follows the "Goldilocks" rule. Too little strain and you may not fully engage your body's repair and growth mechanisms. Too much strain and you'll set yourself up for injury. If you're in pain for days after a workout and unable to stay on your exercise schedule, you're likely pushing too hard. Aim for the level of exercise intensity that is "just right."

Recovery time is also critical in exercise. During a workout, you are not building strength and resiliency of muscles, tendons, ligaments, and cartilage. Anabolic and inflammation-resolving factors activate during recovery. Coaches and trainers are now quite aware of the need for cycles of exercise that include periods of rest. Ask any baseball pitching coach and you'll get a detailed explanation of the maximum pitch counts they allow for their athletes. Recovery isn't just important for professional pitchers and athletes. Recovery is for everyone of all fitness levels trying to build strength and repair tendons, ligaments, and cartilage.

Exercise Resolves Chronic Inflammatory Disease

The ability of exercise to resolve chronic inflammation is undeniable and supported by multiple studies. A compelling example of the benefits of exercise involves patients with a chronic inflammatory muscle disease called myositis.[4] People with this condition are often debilitated by weakness and muscle pain. They're traditionally treated with strong immune suppressants such as corticosteroids and told to avoid exercise. This advice was based on the inflammatory cytokines that are released during exercise and the concern that acute inflammation would worsen their myositis. Imposing exercise limitations for people suffering from chronic muscle inflammation makes sense. Unfortunately, these traditional recommendations underestimate the power of exercise to turn on the body's natural inflammation-resolving factors. Several studies show improvements from exercise, such as strength training, for patients with myositis. With an exercise program, markers of muscle inflammation and pain *decrease* over time for people with myositis, and their strength improves.[5] Medications do not show results for this group that are as impressive.

Some of the strength and health benefits of a workout are reduced by medications such as NSAIDs. Recall from Chapter 3, Current Osteoarthritis Treatments, that NSAIDs block COX enzymes and the synthesis of prostaglandins. Reducing inflammatory prostaglandins decreases pain. It also limits the recruitment of white blood cells to the area and prevents the macrophage transition to an M2 cell. Without the inflammation-resolving activities of the M2 macrophage, protein and collagen production decrease and muscle growth is impaired.[6] The importance of the macrophage in driving exercise benefits is further supported by a research study that reduced the number

of macrophages in blood circulation before exercise in laboratory animals. When macrophage numbers dwindled, so did
muscle growth.[7] The negative effects of NSAIDs are most significant when used before exercise. If you're taking an NSAID
around the time of exercise, it is best to take it after your workout, not before. A shorter work out *without* an NSAID is more
beneficial (and safer) than a longer one *with* this medication.

Exercise not only improves chronic pain from OA or myositis,
but it also helps to recover from acute injuries. If you've had a
sprain or sports injury, you were likely advised to rest the painful
area. There is even an acronym for this: RICE, indicating rest, ice,
compression, and elevation. Rest is often needed immediately
after an injury and you should ask your doctor or physical therapist when it is safe to return to exercise cautiously. However, prolonged, complete rest can increase the levels of MMP enzymes in
tendons, ligaments, and cartilage and worsen damage.

One particularly compelling study demonstrates the potential harms of prolonged rest. The researchers analyzed MRIs
of knee cartilage before and after ankle fracture surgery. You
might wonder, "Why look at the knee when the knee wasn't
injured?" The researchers knew that patients would be on
crutches after these fractures, and their knee (on the side with
the injured ankle) would experience minimal weight bearing
and motion for several weeks. When the investigators compared the before and after MRIs, they found that the unin-
jured knee lost significant cartilage thickness.[8] Prolonged rest
for patients' ankles (and therefore their knees) decreased the
health of their knees.

There are times when complete rest is necessary, such as
after a fracture or surgery. For more minor injuries, it's a good
idea to resume activity as soon as your medical or surgical team

Healthy Function

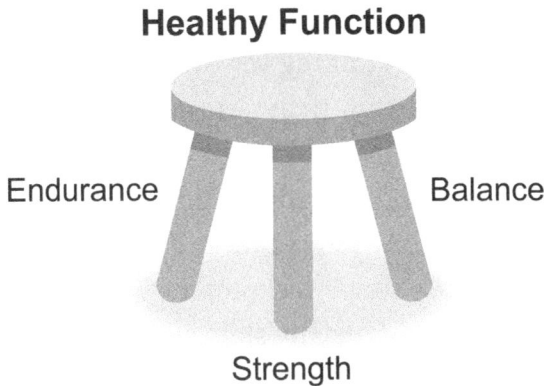

Endurance   Balance

Strength

Figure 8.1. Contributions to healthy function.

says it is safe to resume exercise and work diligently with your physical therapist or trainer to exercise safely.

The Pillars of Exercise

The three pillars of exercise are endurance, strength, and balance. These skills are the foundation of health throughout your life and are even more critical as you age. With endurance, you'll be able to take walks in your seventies, eighties, and nineties that improve the health of your joints. With strength, you'll be able to lift your grandchild or great-grandchild. With balance, you can move and lift with stability and confidence. In addition to offering functional benefits, these fitness pillars also reduce pain and stiffness if you have OA.[9] Together, the three pillars lead to long-term healthy function and vitality (Figure 8.1).

Endurance Training

One of the primary ways to improve endurance is through aerobic training. Aerobic workouts, regardless of type, share an expected outcome of increased heart rate. To better assess the intensity of different styles of endurance training, exercise scientists often classify aerobic work into distinct zones. It might be evident that running for thirty minutes requires significantly greater exertion than casually strolling for the same period. However, other comparisons may be less easy to make. Is swimming more vigorous than jogging? What about Zumba versus basketball? Using heart rate as a guide makes categorizing the intensity of various workouts easier.

Exercise intensities typically start at Zone 1 (a casual walk), progress to Zone 2 (a brisk walk or slow jog), and end up at the out-of-breath Zone 5. A Zone 5 activity pushes you to near maximum heart rate. In Zone 5, you are exercising at an intensity that can only be sustained for a few minutes. At Zone 5, you become quickly exhausted and are unable to speak. Zone 5 is not where you want to be when starting an exercise routine. It is also important to note that in Zone 5, your body is no longer using mitochondria efficiently, which you learned about in Chapter 4, How Nerves (Mal)Function. You're breaking down glucose for its fast-release ATP and building up lactic acid in the muscles. Although there are benefits of Zone 5 exercise, mitochondria are probably better trained with more prolonged bouts of lower-intensity exercise.

If you're dealing with OA pain, you want to spend most of your exercise time doing Zone 2 activities, such as brisk walking. With this moderate-intensity exercise, you are not only less likely to be injured, but you are also strengthening cartilage, tendons, and ligaments. A meta-analysis of 17 studies has confirmed the power of aerobic exercises, such as walking, to improve pain and endurance in patients with OA.[10]

Aerobic exercise not only improves symptoms, but it also appears to slow OA development as measured by X-ray.[11] These benefits come from two sources. The first benefit is

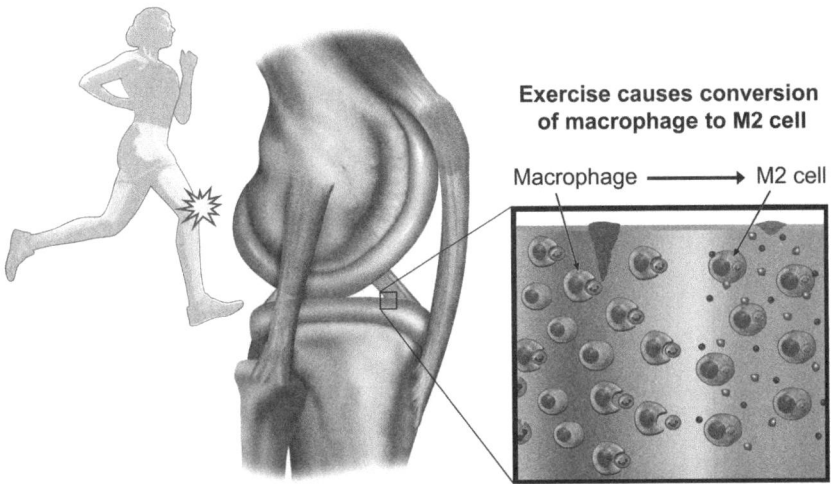

Figure 8.2. Exercise effect on immune cells: Exercise stimulates the immune system, leading to M2 cell production of anabolic factors and mechanical nutrient flow to chondrocytes (cartilage cells).

exercise-induced immune stimulation, the transition of joint macrophages to M2 cells, and the subsequent release of anabolic cytokines and growth factors (Figure 8.2). The second benefit stems from applying weight to your knees and other joints with each step of your walk. The repeated mild to moderate impacts move synovial fluid in and out of the cartilage that has no direct blood supply. With each step, the cartilage cells receive the nutritive factors your body has made. Chondrocytes (the cartilage cells introduced in Chapter 1, Joint Anatomy and the Myth of "Wear and Tear") become more resilient and better able to produce collagen, proteoglycan, and other cartilage matrix materials that restore joint health.

What about more demanding exercises, such as running? In this situation, it is important to consider individual factors (level of fitness, prior injuries) and the dose and intensity of the attempted exercise. Recreational running does not appear to damage cartilage. This conclusion is supported by a 2023 meta-analysis published in *The Orthopedic Journal of Sports Medicine* in which the effect of running on cartilage health and thickness was measured. Those who ran had just as much knee cartilage as those who didn't.[12] So, to keep joints healthy, take a brisk walk daily. If you like to run for aerobic fitness, rest assured that you can do this without undoing any of the benefits from your walking. Don't fear "wear and tear." Pursue "exercise and improve."

Strength Training

You may think of strength training as something younger athletes do. Perhaps you have an image of a high school or college football team in the weight room, preparing for the upcoming season. It's time to put that stereotype to rest. Although weight training is essential for nearly everyone, people over sixty may benefit the most. In your sixties, muscle loss speeds up, leading to frailty in later life if you do nothing about it. Strength training slows muscle loss and significantly improves the stability of joints. Strength exercise also decreases long-term levels of inflammatory cytokines such as IL-1 and TNF and increases beneficial molecules such as hyaluronic acid. This combination of greater stability, decreased chronic inflammation, and improved joint lubrication can significantly reduce pain.

If you're new to strength training, find a trainer or physical therapist to help guide you. They can help you build a program that will progressively improve strength while minimizing the chances of injury. A strength routine should be challenging but not overwhelming for your muscles and joints. Choosing a gym where the weight room is visited with individuals of all ages can assure that you will get the instruction and support you need.

Balance Training

Standing on two feet is a complex balancing task. It requires rapid, coordinated interactions between the nerves from your limbs, inner ears, and eyes. These multiple inputs are processed continuously in your brain and relayed back to the muscles of the hips, legs, and feet to keep you upright. This finely tuned system is thrown off if any part of this system misfires. People with vertigo know this all too well. Those with peripheral neuropathy from diabetes, chemotherapy, or other metabolic disorders also experience impaired balance. Their brains receive incomplete signals from their feet and legs and struggle to coordinate the fine muscle movements needed to maintain balance and avoid falls.

The balance systems in the body can be trained and improved. Some of these training exercises are best guided by physical therapists. Others can be done on your own. Walking with a friend improves balance, especially when good conversation pulls your mental focus away from each step and adds to the task's complexity. Standing on one leg is also an activity that can be done at home. Just don't forget to have a chair in front of you to prevent falls. As you navigate on uneven surfaces or balance on one side, you train the coordination between peripheral nerves, muscles, inner ears, eyes, and brain.

Additional beneficial skills are learned with yoga, tai chi, and related practices. These mind-body practices offer an excellent combination of balance training, strength building, and meditation. Yoga, a 5,000-year-old physical/spiritual practice from northern India, has an estimated 35 million practitioners in the US and its popularity continues to grow. Yoga has been shown to improve pain, physical function, and quality of life for OA patients.[13] Yoga works well and quickly, offering benefits after only a few weeks. Yoga is a wonderful complement to a strengthening and walking program if you're trying to reduce your pain and improve your function with OA.

Tai chi is a Taoist-based ancient martial art focused on establishing equilibrium in body motion and nature. The exercises combine slow, purposeful weight shifting and balance activities with controlled breathing and meditation. Tai chi is now practiced by almost 4 million people in the US. It has been shown to significantly improve balance, function, and pain in people with knee OA.[14] Some individuals with joint pain find tai chi easier than yoga, although this depends on the joints involved and the style of tai chi. Tai chi has been shown to provide similar benefits to physical therapy with additional positive effects on depression and anxiety.[15] If you have joint pain, it is worth exploring these ancient practices for their potential benefits of balance, strength, and mental health.

Exercise for a Lifetime

Everyone starts at a different place with exercise. You might currently be able to run, bike, or play tennis daily. Or you may struggle to complete a short walk because of joint pain. Regardless of where you are, the important thing is to find an activity that you *can* do. If walking is too painful, try an exercise bike. If the exercise bike is too difficult, consider aqua therapy. A workout in the water allows for joint motion and strengthening under nearly weightless conditions. It's a wonderful, gentle exercise for painful knees and hips. If you don't like the water, perhaps tai chi is a good fit. Start somewhere and then build on that routine. Keep an exercise diary. If you can walk for only 10 minutes or do tai chi for 15 minutes, that's okay. Write that number down.

If getting started is a problem for you, consider getting help. Seek assistance from a physical therapist or trainer. Physical therapists and trainers have expertise in body mechanics and can also observe your gait while walking, your form while lifting a weight, or your swing with a racquet. They will help you develop a program that builds endurance, strength, and balance while minimizing the risks of injury.

Return to your initial written number intermittently as you progress with your exercise program. Some people like to track their exercise daily. Keep in mind, though, that there will be fluctuations in your exercise tolerance depending on many factors. A more strenuous workout on Wednesday may lead to reduced performance on Thursday. That's okay. Treat Thursday as a recovery day. The goal is slow, steady progress over weeks, not days. Elite athletes understand this. If they're training for a competition and miss a week due to illness, they know not to accelerate their training schedule too rapidly, or they'll find themselves injured.

Over the course of weeks or months, you may notice your knee hurts a little less during your walk and may not be as sore the day after your walks. You might find yourself taking less ibuprofen or pain medication in the evening. You may notice you're sleeping a bit better at night, and your energy is improved during the day. Research indicates that you will enjoy these benefits if you remain persistent and give yourself time.

Exercise is a regenerative therapy. The inflammation/recovery cycles of an exercise program activate immune-based repair mechanisms that manufacture the proteins, collagen, and other substances needed to restore health to muscles, tendons, ligaments, and cartilage. These benefits not only occur locally, but at distant sites where pain-relieving growth factors and cytokines are carried through the bloodstream too. Walking will certainly help your knee pain. It may also improve the arthritis pain in your other joints.

In the next chapter, I explain how exercise is also the foundation of nerve health and introduce you to a tiny particle—the exosome—that carries out many of these beneficial effects.

Takeaways

1 Exercise stimulates the immune system to release anabolic and inflammation-resolving factors.
2. It's best to cycle exercise with periods of recovery, giving the body time for repair mechanisms to work.
3. The three pillars of exercise (aerobic endurance, strength, and balance) form a foundation to promote long-term health.

Chapter 9

Exercise, Exosomes, and Reversing Neuropathy

After surgery, Marcus experienced significant benefits from his walking and strength program. His sciatica pain faded, and his function progressively improved. He returned to work, resumed activities with his family, and restarted (occasional) backyard projects. Surgery and injection removed the pressure on his nerves. Exercise activated the mechanisms to resolve his pain.

Exercise Improves Sensation and Pain

The improvements Marcus experienced from exercise aren't surprising. Physical therapy, strengthening, and walking have been shown to reduce acute and chronic sciatica pain and improve recovery after spine surgery.[1] Stronger back and abdominal muscles support the spine and its motion. As spine mechanics improve, the exiting spinal nerves experience less compression and, therefore, less pain. Enhanced mechanics is not the only reason sciatica improves with exercise. Exercise directly restores nerve health. These improvements are seen not only in the sciatic nerve but also in the peripheral nerves of the feet and hands.

Recall from Chapter 4, How Nerves (Mal)Function, that approximately one-half of the individuals who have diabetes or have received chemotherapy drugs, such as paclitaxel, experience neuropathy. They have numbness, tingling, and frequent pain from damage to the long peripheral nerves. This neuropathy pain can be debilitating. Medications can help some individuals, but they're not effective for all and frequently cause side effects. Fortunately, exercises such as walking and balance training can significantly reduce the pain.[2] The benefits are further magnified when strength training is added to the workout.

Exercise also improves nerve function. Even a short, eight-week program of low-to-moderate-intensity treadmill walking (equivalent to Zone 1–2) can restore sensation in the feet of those with diabetic neuropathy.[3] The return of nerve activity provides multiple health benefits. In addition to reducing pain, restored nerve function allows an individual to sense their steps more accurately, especially on uneven surfaces. Improved foot sensation provides greater feedback to the brain, re-establishing balance and coordination circuits. Better balance helps people to avoid falls, injuries, and fractures. These exercise-based improvements in sensory function, pain, and health in individuals with neuropathy don't take years. They take only weeks.

Exercise Can Prevent Neuropathy

Exercise may be an even more powerful tool in the *prevention* of neuropathy. In 2018, the results from a multicenter exercise study in 355 patients with breast, colon, lung, and other cancers were published.[4] Before these patients started chemotherapy, they were assessed for neuropathy symptoms (numbness and tingling in feet or hands). They were then given pedometers and randomly assigned to either an exercise program or standard care, which did not include exercise instructions. The exercisers were given resistance bands and a walking prescription. They were instructed on how to perform the resistance exercises, increasing the size and tension of these giant rubber bands as tolerated. In addition, this group was coached to increase their walking time progressively. After the six-week study, the differences in walking duration between the two groups weren't dramatic. The exercise group walked, on average, 650 more steps per day. Nonetheless, this modest increase in steps, combined with the resistance band activities, significantly improved nerve health. Fewer exercisers developed neuropathy from their chemotherapy than patients in the other group. And those exercisers who did develop neuropathy had less severe symptoms.

Exercise's long-term protective effects were also tested in a four-year study in Rome, Italy. Researchers evaluated the nerve function, weight, and metabolic state of participants with diabetes but no neuropathy.[5] Metabolism was assessed by measuring HbA1c (a measure of long-term glucose control), lipids, and body fat. Their nerve function was assessed by testing skin sensation and nerve conduction velocities.

Nerve conduction velocity testing is a technique that has been used for decades to measure the speed and function of nerves. During this test, electrodes are placed on the skin at two different points of a peripheral nerve where neuropathy is suspected. A pulse of electricity is then delivered to one of the electrodes. The nerve conduction velocity is the time it takes for the electrical signal to travel from the electrical pulse electrode to the measurement electrode. A peripheral nerve affected by diabetes, chemotherapy, or compression frequently slows down and shows a decreased velocity. If the damage is severe, the nerve may not conduct any electrical impulse at all. Nerve conduction velocities can be a valuable tool to assess the functional state of a peripheral nerve and to measure any changes over time.

The people in the Rome study were then randomly assigned to either an exercise (brisk treadmill walking) group or a standard care group for four years. At the end of the study, researchers reassessed participants' nerve conduction velocities, skin sensation, and metabolic state. Thirty percent of the nonexercisers developed neuropathy symptoms, and the group's nerve velocities slowed. On the other hand, only six percent of the exercisers developed neuropathy. More remarkably, when nerve conduction velocities were evaluated in the exercise group, there was an increase in velocity. Not only did exercise prevent neuropathy, but it also restored nerve function in many of the individuals with diabetes.

When I read this study, I assumed that the improvements in nerve function reflected improved metabolic health in the exercisers. This was a reasonable assumption given that exercise is known to lower blood glucose, reduce weight, and reduce the metabolic drivers of neuropathy. However, when glucose levels, weight, and other metabolic measurements were assessed at the end of the study, there was no difference between the exercisers and nonexercisers. It wasn't the metabolic improvements that restored nerve function in these individuals with diabetes. There was something else—an unmeasured factor.

Exercise Helps Nerves Regrow

So far, in this chapter, I've discussed how scientists can test the *function* of peripheral nerves through skin sensation and nerve conduction velocities. With the aid of a microscope, the *structure* of peripheral nerves can also be assessed. This process requires a small skin biopsy (typically from the foot or ankle where neuropathy symptoms occur). Biopsied skin is soaked in a stain that binds to the small peripheral nerves. When examined under a microscope, the nerves light up. In people with neuropathy, some of these nerves die back. Others appear swollen and sick. The mitochondria (the cell's remarkable energy battery discussed in Chapter 4) of these nerve cells don't function well. Cell proteins are also abnormal.

With the microscope, scientists can count nerves and calculate nerve fiber density. Researchers used nerve fiber density testing to assess the effects of a ten-week exercise program for patients with diabetic neuropathy. Before the study participants began their exercise program, they had skin biopsies taken and researchers counted their nerve fibers. Participants then began to exercise. The program included aerobic workouts (moderate-intensity bicycle or treadmill exercise) combined with strength work. At the end of the ten weeks, many participants demonstrated increased nerve fiber density. Exercise had regrown their nerves. Even better, their pain also decreased.[6]

Nerve fiber density calculations have also been used to assess the preventive effects of exercise on neuropathy. Researchers from the University of Utah studied 100 patients with diabetes who hadn't yet experienced any neuropathy symptoms. The patients were randomly assigned to either lifestyle counseling (diet and exercise) or a supervised exercise program (equivalent to Zone 2 with added strength training). Researchers took skin biopsies and calculated nerve fiber densities at the beginning of the study. The researchers' first discovery was that, although none of the participants had a clinical neuropathy diagnosis, many already had decreased nerve fiber density. The loss of small peripheral nerves in the skin appeared to proceed the decrease in skin sensation observed by traditional testing.

Nerve fiber density calculations were repeated at the end of the 12-month study. The lifestyle counseling group experienced limited change. In contrast, the exercise group demonstrated significant improvement in nerve fiber density and a trend toward protection from neuropathy.[7] The study revealed that exercise restores small peripheral nerves to health and likely prevents the onset of clinical nerve dysfunction.

Exercise's Tiny Particle: The Exosome

You now know that exercise is a powerful tool in preventing and treating neuropathy. In Chapter 7, Fats and Plant Colors to Resolve Inflammation, you also learned that exercise can turn on the healing cascade by releasing bursts of inflammatory cytokines such as IL-6. Immune stimulation, however, doesn't completely explain the nerve improvements from a brisk walk or strength training. The unmeasured factor delivering many of these benefits is likely a tiny particle, about one-tenth the size of mitochondria.

This particle, the exosome, was discovered in the 1980s and was initially thought to be a waste removal system for cells. At the time, this conclusion was logical. These fluid-filled particles were seen packing up various cellular materials and releasing them outside the cell. These vesicles appeared to be removing the cell's garbage just like you take out your household garbage. In recent years, the scientific community has realized that it greatly underestimated the important role of the exosome in restoring cell health. Exosomes aren't taking out the trash. They're carefully preparing materials to share with other cells, such as neurons, in an elaborate cell-to-cell communication system.

Exosomes are produced by all cells and found throughout our bodies. They are in our blood, joint fluid, spinal fluid, cartilage cells, neurons, and Schwann cells, and they are an important component of breast milk. Exosomes carry diverse cargo, such as proteins, DNA, RNA, and a particular type of RNA called micro-RNA (miRNA), which I will introduce in the next chapter. Exosomes regulate immune cells, nerve function, and the resolution of pain.[8] Their release increases during stress, high temperature, low oxygen, and acid buildup—conditions the body commonly produces with exercise. Exercise of all intensities produces exosomes. A brisk walk will release exosomes as well as a high-intensity workout. Exosomes deliver many of the benefits of exercise for nerve function, muscle strength, and even cartilage health.[9]

Exosomes are created by cells. First, the cell's membrane folds inward, forming a protective bubble called an endosome. The endosome then travels inside the cell, gathering various proteins, DNA, RNA, and miRNA. The endosome double-wraps this cargo into smaller protective bubbles called vesicles. In the final step, the endosome with its vesicles is sent back to the cell membrane. The endosome fuses with the membrane and releases the tiny vesicles to the outside, now called exosomes (Figure 9.1).

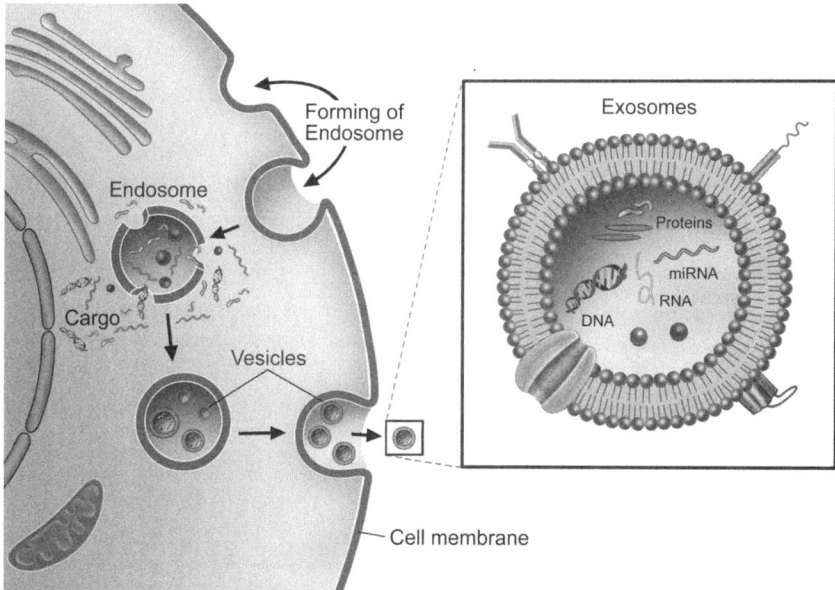

Figure 9.1. Exosome creation: An endosome forms and gathers proteins, DNA, RNA, and miRNA inside the cell. The cargo is then double-wrapped into smaller bubbles called vesicles. Once released outside of the cell, the vesicles are called exosomes.

Exosomes carry and protect fragile cargo on the journey to distant targets such as peripheral nerves, cartilage, and muscle. The exosome coating prevents enzymes from breaking down RNA, miRNA, and other vulnerable components in transit. When exosomes reach their target cells, they enter and release their rich contents. Exosomes and their cargo can significantly change the behavior of the recipient cell, including its genetic activity and protein production.[10]

It's essential to remember that exosomes are only as good as their contents. The quality of the contents depends on the source cell and the conditions in which the cell lives. Exosomes are like delivery packages you might receive at your house or apartment. Imagine that, one day, you arrive home to see that you and your neighbor both have packages of garden seeds sitting at your front door. The packages look identical and contain the same number of tomato, basil, and jalapeño pepper seeds. The package similarities are remarkable, given that they're produced by different companies in different regions of the US. You and your neighbor plant those seeds in similar pots with similar soil on adjacent porches with similar sun exposure and watering schedules. A few weeks later, on a lovely Saturday afternoon, you go outside to transplant your seedlings in the garden and see that your neighbor is doing the same. Your neighbor's tomatoes and peppers are shooting up with firm stalks. Her basil is already lush and green. You look down at your seedlings. Many of the pots are empty; the seeds didn't germinate. The plants that did grow look sickly, and some leaves have already yellowed. You sigh in resignation, knowing it won't be a good year for your vegetable garden. You're also puzzled. The packages appeared nearly identical. How were the contents and functions of those packages so markedly different?

The function of exosomes similarly depends on the sources and cargo. Exosomes derived from exhausted cells may have no effect, and those from an arthritic knee may do more harm than good. Conversely, exosomes produced in the blood following exercise reflect the beneficial stresses of a workout. They contain proteins and multiple factors that can promote muscle growth, nerve health, and pain reduction.

Exosomes Protect Nerves

Diseases such as diabetes and toxins such as chemotherapy reduce mitochondrial function in neurons. Without optimal mitochondrial activity, the transport of growth factors and proteins diminishes. Neurons—especially those with long axons—can't keep up their high-voltage activities and begin to malfunction. Nerve conduction velocities slow, neurons die back, and nerve fiber density decreases.

In addition to energy failure, dysfunctional mitochondria also leak charged protons and electrons into the cell. These charged molecules can change the shape of proteins, rendering them ineffective or unusable. Loose, high-energy particles in the cell can also damage DNA, increasing the risk of cancer or cell death. Malfunctioning mitochondria cause persistent damage and chronic inflammation unless they are removed.

Fortunately, exosomes provide multiple repair mechanisms for the neuron's mitochondria. The release of these exosomes during exercise bathes the neuron with multiple protective vesicles. Exercise also improves the quality of the exosome cargo, packing them with proteins and miRNA that stimulate nerve repair. Exercise and exosomes are intimately linked. Exosomes deliver many of the benefits of a workout.

One of the repair mechanisms that exosomes support is mitochondrial autophagy, the recycling of damaged mitochondria presented in Chapter 4. As autophagy increases, damage and chronic inflammation from leaking mitochondria diminishes. The health and function of the neuron improve. Exosomes also boost the manufacturing process that builds new mitochondria. This increase in mitochondrial numbers restores the supply of ATP, the adenosine triphosphate molecule that provides energy for all the active processes in living cells. With reestablished energy supplies, neurons resume transport mechanisms for proteins and growth factors up and down their long axons. Neurons re-energize and power the electrical transmission that allows us to feel the ground, regain balance, and reduce the risks of falls. The peripheral nerve starts working again.

Exosomes additionally regulate immune cell function. They promote the transition of macrophages to M2 cells in the nervous system that you learned about in Chapter 6, Igniting the Immune System to Heal, releasing growth factors, anabolic cytokines, and inflammation-resolving lipids. These immune cell changes reduce chronic inflammation and decrease neuropathy pain.[11] Exosomes and their cargo deliver these protective functions to neurons throughout the body. Exercise and the exosomes it releases repair mitochondria, improve energy stores, speed up nerve velocity, reduce chronic inflammation, and reduce neuropathy pain.

There is a tremendous interest in using manufactured exosomes to treat multiple degenerative conditions such as osteoarthritis and neuropathy. Unfortunately, there is not yet a commercially available, FDA-approved source of these exosomes in the US. The FDA has also shuttered several companies that produced these exosomes because they had not undergone the necessary quality and safety testing. But people still have access to safe and effective exosomes. We produce billions of them with every workout. Exosomes are also naturally produced with the regenerative therapies that I describe in future chapters.[12]

The evidence is clear that exosomes play a critical role in restoring mitochondrial and nerve function. In the next chapter, you'll learn that exosome contents are also powerful epigenetic tools, able to reprogram DNA function and even turn back the aging clock.

Takeaways

1 Exercise improves nerve function and reduces pain.
2 Exercise releases exosomes that carry protective proteins, DNA, RNA, and miRNA.
3 Exosomes and their cargo promote mitochondrial repair, increase energy supplies, and reduce chronic nerve inflammation.

Chapter 10

Epigenetics and Aging

Neurons, cartilage cells, and macrophages have very different functions, but they have one thing in common. These cells (and all the other nonreproductive cells) in your body have the same DNA. What allows each cell type to develop vastly different functions and appearances is "epigenetics." Epigenetics determines whether a cell becomes a neuron or a macrophage. It also controls the resiliency and health of cells throughout their lifespan. Epigenetics is the software that runs your genetic hardware.

Like software, epigenetics can malfunction. It can also be updated and restored under the right conditions. Although epigenetics doesn't change your genes, it turns genes up, down, on, and off. Epigenetics regulates the cytokines, growth factors, and enzymes such as MMP that I introduced in Chapter 2, How to Damage Cartilage, significantly affecting (positively or negatively) the development of osteoarthritis (OA).[1] These same epigenetic mechanisms regulate the body's response to injury and the risks of developing chronic pain.[2] Epigenetic regulation isn't limited to painful conditions. It also affects the risk of cancer, cardiac disease, and neurologic disorders, such as Alzheimer's dementia and Parkinson's disease.[3]

Epigenetics additionally drives the aging process. As cells develop, they acquire a specific epigenetic "signature" that makes one cell a neuron and another a cartilage cell. This signature continues throughout adult life but can erode over time, like a vinyl music record. When first pressed, a record has distinct grooves that transmit the original music with high fidelity. With frequent use, however, the record grooves wear down. The music still plays, but the guitar riffs and vocals may not be as distinct or powerful as they once were.

Similar to a vinyl record, a cell also loses the "grooves" of its epigenetic signature over time. This loss of cellular high fidelity was demonstrated with a series of experiments published in 2023 by scientists at Harvard and collaborating institutions.[4] These researchers showed that as epigenetic grooves erode, cell functions slow down, mitochondria malfunction, and cell damage begins to appear. The cell may continue to live but starts secreting inflammatory cytokines that affect its health and the health of neighboring cells. The good news is that these changes are not irreversible. They are not written in the genetic code. They are *epi*-genetic—layered on top of the genes. To better understand how to restore the epigenetics of your cells and improve OA or neuropathy pain, I need to first explain how these mechanisms actually work.

Epigenetics: Controlling Proteins Made from DNA

The human body generates about 100,000 different kinds of proteins. These building block molecules, made from nitrogen-containing amino acids you absorb from your diet, make up the mitochondria, nerves, tendons, ligaments, cartilage, and muscles. They allow humans to think, move, fight infection, and recover from injury. They control nearly every process in the body and keep people alive. The curious thing about the 100,000 different proteins is that they're made from only about 25,000 DNA genes. Each DNA gene segment can generate multiple different kinds of proteins through various splicing techniques and intermediate steps.

To make a protein, the gene first has to be copied. Genes don't exist as single strands of DNA but in segments. Mechanisms in the body copy these segments and splice them together to make messenger RNA (mRNA). For instance, if DNA has sequences for A-B-C-D, it can make an mRNA with sequences of A-B-C, A-B-D, or various other combinations. Splicing can create multiple different versions of mRNA from a single gene.

The mRNA then serves as a blueprint for the next step, which is the assembly of amino acids into chains that form proteins. The human body uses 20 different types of amino acids to manufacture all of its proteins. Amino acids contain a central carbon atom and nitrogen (the amino group). What makes each amino acid distinct are the various side groups attached to the carbon atom. The side group defines the shape and function of the amino acid and, therefore, of the final protein.

Proteins are extraordinarily diverse in size. Some, like collagen, are small and made of only 20 amino acids. Others, like muscle proteins, are huge, using as many as 3,500 amino acids. This sequence of events—(a) copying and splicing DNA to mRNA and then (b) using mRNA as a blueprint to assemble amino acids into proteins—defines the function of every cell in your body.

Epigenetics controls these steps. It defines which DNA genes are chosen for copying and how the mRNA is spliced. Even after the mRNA is made, epigenetics determines if this messenger survives to make a protein or is destroyed before carrying out its task. Epigenetics defines the kinds of proteins manufactured and, therefore, the cell's behavior, personality, and aging. It does so through three main mechanisms:

1. histone protein modifications,

2. DNA methylation, and

3. microRNAs (miRNAs).

Histone Protein Modification: Wrapping for Your DNA

The nucleus contains all of the cell's chromosomes, which encode the genetic material. Inside the nucleus, DNA is wrapped tightly around proteins called histones (Figure 10.1). Histone proteins serve as structural support for the long DNA strands. If a cell's DNA were unwound, it would be more than six feet long. DNA's tightly wound structure is necessary to fit all of the DNA into the cell's tiny nucleus.

In addition to providing structural support, histones also play a crucial functional role. When DNA is wrapped tightly around histone proteins, DNA is hidden from the machinery that copies DNA to mRNA. The tighter the DNA binding to histones, the more the DNA is hidden and "silenced." Epigenetics controls this process by adding or subtracting molecules to the sides of histone proteins. If molecules are added, the DNA loosens and unwinds, allowing it to be copied to mRNA. If molecules are removed, the DNA rewraps itself tightly. Histone protein modification is a dynamic process affected by lifestyle factors such as diet, sleep, and exercise. The epigenetic mechanisms control the copying of DNA to mRNA.

Sirtuins are a group of important histone protein regulators. They remove molecules from histones, causing the DNA to wrap even more tightly. Their activities silence the associated DNA gene. Sirtuins carry out multiple functions throughout the body. They are richly supplied in glial cells, such as Schwann cells, that surround peripheral nerves. Sirtuins regulate the release of exosomes that Schwann cells transfer to neurons, especially during stress. Sirtuins also turn on mitochondrial autophagy (discussed in Chapter 4, How Nerves [Mal] Function), recycling mitochondrial parts and restoring energy supplies to nerves and cartilage.[5] Sirtuin proteins control the synthesis of multiple cartilage components, such as collagen

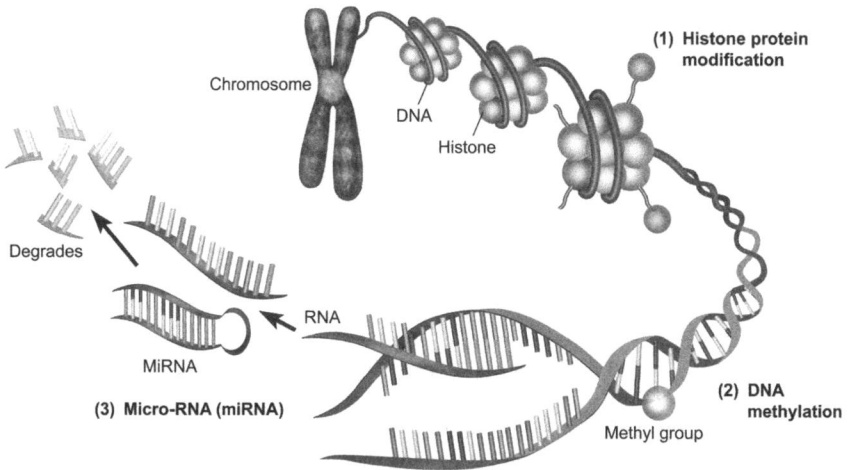

Figure 10.1. Mechanisms of epigenetic regulation: (1) Histone protein modification: Molecules added to histones loosen the DNA and make it available for mRNA copying; (2) DNA methylation: Methyl groups added to DNA prevent the copying of DNA to mRNA; (3) miRNA: miRNAs bind to mRNA and prevent the assembly of proteins.

and proteoglycan, and can reduce the production of damaging MMP enzymes.[6] This combination of effects is vital for cartilage preservation. Sirtuins turn on protective mechanisms for nerves, cartilage, and nearly all of the cells in the body.

Sirtuin proteins have also attracted attention recently because of their potential benefits for human longevity. These proteins—when released under stress—signal cells to stop growing and to start conserving resources. Sirtuins not only turn on recycling systems such as autophagy but also generate protective proteins and silence unnecessary cell activities. These housecleaning activities help cells survive in times of hardship and build resilience.

Multiple kinds of stresses can turn on these sirtuin proteins. Fasting and calorie restriction activate sirtuins. Intermittent heat stress, such as a sauna, also stimulates the production of these sirtuin proteins. The most potent stimulus for sirtuin activity, however, is exercise.[7] Exercise, especially strength training and higher-intensity workouts, turns on short- and long-term sirtuin proteins. The combination of sirtuin-based housecleaning activities and the anabolic and tissue-building effects of exercise growth factors restore the health of neurons, cartilage, muscles, and tendons. The benefits of sirtuins are epigenetic. They're not changing genes. They're changing how genes behave.

DNA Methylation: Defining Your Biologic Age

Another powerful epigenetic tool is the addition of methyl groups directly to DNA. Methyl groups are stable molecules consisting of a carbon atom bound to hydrogens. When methyl groups bind to DNA, the process is called methylation. The methyl groups prevent the DNA from being copied to mRNA, effectively silencing the gene. In this way, methylation produces long-lasting epigenetic changes. DNA methylation occurs in all species and is critical in embryonic development and growth. Each cell type has a different DNA methylation "signature" that drives its specialization and function. A cartilage cell, a neuron, and a macrophage each have a different methylation pattern. These methyl groups turn different genes on and off, allowing different cell types to develop distinct appearances and roles.

Although methylation is generally stable in adulthood, like those vinyl records mentioned earlier, methylation loses its grooves over time. These erosion patterns have been extensively studied and can now be used to calculate the biological age of cells. DNA methylation changes in predictable patterns with the number of years a person is alive. It also changes with lifestyle, exposure to toxins, and chronic stress.[8] For instance, DNA methylation of identical twins is nearly the same at birth. But twin's methylation patterns diverge with different life experiences and exposures. If one of the twins begins to smoke tobacco, the methylation patterns of that twin's cells quickly change. Although born on the same day, the smoking twin acquires an older epigenetic age than the other twin. Methylation patterns reflect biological age and can increasingly predict susceptibility to degenerative diseases.

Methylation patterns and epigenetic age can also improve with healthy lifestyle changes. The ability to reduce biological age was shown in a study published by authors at the Institute for Functional Medicine and several collaborating universities in 2021.[9] These researchers tested the epigenetic age of 43 individuals who agreed to have their DNA methylation patterns analyzed before and after an eight-week diet and lifestyle intervention. The volunteers were randomly assigned to two groups. One group received an intervention of daily exercise, adequate sleep, relaxation training, and a vegetable/nutrient-enriched diet. The other group received no treatment. Not surprisingly, those who received no intervention saw little change in DNA methylation patterns.

Conversely, the DNA methylation age of those who received the lifestyle intervention was reduced by over three years. They grew epigenetically younger. This research study and others demonstrate that although methylation patterns of cells may erode over time, these changes are not written in stone (or the genetic code).

miRNA: Changing How Cells Behave

The third epigenetic mechanism involves a special kind of RNA called microRNAs (miRNAs). miRNAs have the unique ability to shut down the assembly line from DNA genes to proteins. Although the acronyms "miRNA" and "mRNA" differ by only one letter, the actions of these RNAs could not be more different. mRNA serves as a blueprint to assemble amino acids into proteins. miRNA does the opposite, halting this process. miRNAs have sequences that match specific mRNAs and bind tightly to them. Once bound, the mRNA is either neutralized or destroyed. miRNAs shut down gene expression (the process of making a functional protein from a gene) in a targeted manner.

miRNAs regulate over 50 percent of gene expression. miRNAs control the immune system, response to injury, function of the healing cascade, and repair systems, such as mitochondrial autophagy. The body makes over a thousand different kinds of miRNA that float throughout joints, nerves, bloodstream, and spinal fluid. To keep track and be able to study them individually, researchers usually describe miRNAs with a number (for example, miRNA-21, miRNA-146, miRNA-124, etc.).

miRNAs additionally regulate the production of collagen in cartilage and have shown the ability to prevent joints from developing osteoarthritis.[10] They can improve pain by increasing levels of inflammation-resolving lipids, such as resolvins, and cytokines, such as IL-10, that you learned about in Chapter 2. Schwann cells also release miRNAs in response to nerve injury. miRNAs guide nerve regrowth and repair, restoring the axons and their protective myelin coating.[11] They work throughout your body and are powerful tools in managing OA and neuropathy.

miRNAs, Exosomes, and Exercise

As powerful as miRNAs are in controlling gene expression and protein production, they are fragile during transport. Unprotected miRNAs in blood and tissues are degraded by enzymes, which break them down into unusable parts. Fortunately, miRNAs have an effective partner for their activities:

the exosomes that you learned about in Chapter 9, Exercise, Exosomes, and Reversing Neuropathy. Exosomes coat miRNAs, delivering over 3,000 different kinds of miRNA throughout your body. When exosomal miRNAs reach their targets, the exosomes directly transfer the epigenetic miRNA molecules to the recipient cell, allowing the miRNAs to alter their behavior. Exosome-delivered miRNAs affect the protein manufacturing and the health of neurons and cartilage cells.

Exosomes and miRNAs make a good team. Without the exosome, miRNAs would be limited in their ability to travel long distances in the body. Without the miRNAs, the effects of exosomes on the target cells would be limited. The benefits of exosome-based miRNA can be impressive. In joints with OA, for instance, exosomes and their miRNAs have been shown to increase the production of collagen proteins, decrease the production of damaging enzymes such as MMP, and promote cartilage growth.[12] Exosomal miRNAs also affect immune cell function. They promote the transition of the macrophage to the M2 cell, producing inflammation-resolving cytokines, growth factors, and lipids.[13] Exosomes and their miRNA cargo are potent tools in treating OA, neuropathy, and the accompanying pain.

In Chapter 9, you learned about exercise's ability to produce exosomes and reduce neuropathy pain. Many of the benefits of these exercise-related exosomes are due to the miRNA content. In addition to increasing the number of exosomes released, exercise enhances the miRNA content of exosomes. The miRNA-packed exosomes improve mitochondrial function and ATP production. They also turn on the machinery that manufactures new mitochondria.[14]

The impact of exercise on exosomes and miRNA quality was recently tested in a study of individuals over 65. In the study, researchers enrolled two different groups of patients. Half were routine exercisers and half were sedentary individuals. Researchers analyzed the exosomes and miRNA of participants both before and after a moderate-intensity exercise session. The differences between the two groups in response to exercise were remarkable. The routine exercisers experienced significant increases in miRNAs linked to muscle growth and tissue repair. The sedentary group saw minimal change.[15] Routine exercise primed growth and repair systems and magnified the benefits of workouts. Exercise is a positive feedback loop, increasing the quantity of exosomes and the quality of their miRNA content. Exercise provides epigenetic benefits.

There is ongoing research into synthetic versions of miRNA for the treatment of degenerative neurologic diseases such as Parkinson's disease, Lou Gehrig's disease, and cardiac disease. There is optimism for these potential treatments. If pharmacology can mimic what nature does, these synthetic miRNAs may prove successful in treating these diseases. Nonetheless, challenges remain. The human body has developed and honed repair mechanisms over the millennia. These repair systems include the interplay of thousands of miRNAs, growth factors, and the immune system. Reproducing those beautifully complex mechanisms in the laboratory won't be an easy task.

You've now learned about the causes of osteoarthritis and neuropathy and the critical role of the immune system in driving a healing response. You also know more about the differences between acute and chronic inflammation and the role of exercise, epigenetics, and the exosome for mitochondrial function and cell health. In upcoming chapters, I introduce and explore regenerative therapies. The foundational knowledge you've gained so far will allow you to understand how these regenerative treatments affect the immune system and how they can relieve pain under the right circumstances. As I start this exploration, I begin on familiar ground—the healing of a wound.

Takeaways

1. Epigenetics controls which DNA genes are copied into proteins and how cells function.
2. Epigenetic methylation patterns of a cell erode with time and exposure to toxins, such as smoking.
3. Exosomes contain epigenetically active miRNAs that can improve joint and nerve health.

Chapter 11

Platelet-Rich Plasma: From Wounds to Joints

Sarah's knee pain lessened with her workouts at the gym and evening walks. Her muscles stayed strong, and her pain was generally under control. But playing sports, such as tennis, remained a struggle. She often ended her matches early because of knee pain and found that stiffness would linger for hours. She switched to pickleball, which was a little better. She was able to play for longer periods and finish her matches. The pain continued, however, affecting her enjoyment of the game and the time with friends. On the advice of one of the other pickleball players, Sarah made a clinic appointment with me, hoping to answer a simple and important question: Was it possible to reduce her pain without surgery?

Sarah and I reviewed her previous knee treatments. She had several weeks of improved pain after an initial corticosteroid injection. A second injection was less effective. We discussed that a third injection was unlikely to be much better and might begin to cause side effects such as cartilage and bone density loss. She had also undergone a hyaluronic acid injection the previous year. The relief it provided lasted longer than the steroids had, but the degree of pain relief wasn't that substantial. She thought (and I agreed) that a hyaluronic acid injection probably wasn't worth repeating. Sarah also shared the discussion with her surgeon, who had recommended that she avoid knee replacement surgery, noting her osteoarthritis (OA) wasn't "bone on bone," and she could still play sports. Sarah remained in orthopedic limbo.

She asked me about a therapy called platelet-rich plasma (PRP). Sarah had heard of this treatment from her pickleball friend, who had experienced an improvement in his knee pain with PRP. Sarah had many questions. What is platelet-rich plasma (PRP)? How does it work? What might it do for her? During that clinic visit, we discussed the basics of PRP, and I gave her some information she could read at home. Our discussion only partially satisfied Sarah's curiosity and desire to know more about this commonly used regenerative therapy.

In this chapter, I'll cover the breadth of what I wanted to share with Sarah during her clinic visit that day. My hope is to provide you, the reader, with a deeper understanding of what platelet-rich plasma (PRP) is and how it works. My explanations will start, unsurprisingly, with the immune cascade and wound healing.

Platelet-Rich Plasma and Wounds

Blood is made up of plasma—a yellowish combination of salt water and proteins—plus platelets and red and white blood cells. The platelets are small—about one-fifth the size of a white blood cell—but numerous. You have billions of platelets. The role platelets play in forming blood clots has been known for over a century. In contrast, their role in promoting healing was unknown until much more recently. In the 1970s, it was discovered that platelets, when activated, released hundreds of growth factors (introduced in Chapter 2, How to Damage Cartilage, and further explained in Chapter 6, Igniting the Immune System to Heal) that could spark the repair of nearby injured tissues. These platelet-based growth factors attracted the attention of Dr. David

Knighton, a surgeon at the University of Minnesota in the 1980s. Knighton was a wound-care specialist, struggling to treat and heal the wounds of individuals with diabetes, vascular disease, and trauma. Often, these lesions would never heal, leading to amputation surgeries. In an effort to heal wounds and preserve limbs, Dr. Knighton began researching the platelet.

Knighton and his research team took blood from their patients with chronic wounds and put it into test tubes. They then added a medication to keep the blood from clotting (an anticoagulant) and spun this blood at high speeds in a centrifuge. When anticoagulated blood is centrifuged, blood cells separate by density. Red blood cells are the densest. They settle to the bottom of the test tube. The white blood cells (leukocytes), such as neutrophils and monocytes, separate next. These leukocytes create a layer called the "buffy coat," named for its pale-yellow color. Above the buffy coat layer of leukocytes is a darker yellow layer of plasma with few cells. During centrifugation, the platelets settle into the buffy coat and the plasma just above the buffy coat (Figure 11.1 on page 132). When these two platelet-rich areas are siphoned off, it is called platelet-rich plasma.

Dr. Knighton removed the platelet-rich plasma layer and added a protein to activate the platelets and release their growth factors. He put this platelet-rich plasma (PRP) and growth factor solution directly on patients' nonhealing areas. Chronic wounds that had been present on average for four years were gone in just over ten weeks. Connective tissues grew and covered the open lesions. Wounds healed. Knighton published these remarkable results in the *Annals of Surgery* in 1986,[1] setting off a wave of enthusiasm for PRP and its wound-healing abilities. The popularity of this blood product quickly spread to other fields, such as oral surgery, where nonhealing wounds are particularly problematic for patients.[2] PRP was also adopted in

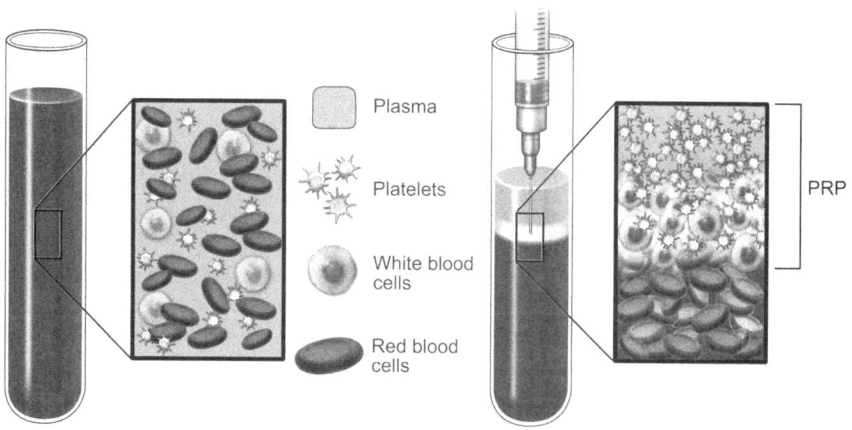

Figure 11.1. Platelet-rich plasma (PRP): Anticoagulated blood is spun in a centrifuge to separate the cells by density. Red blood cells are the densest and settle to the bottom. Above the red blood cells is the "buffy coat" that contains leukocytes, such as neutrophils and monocytes. Above the buffy coat is the plasma. Platelets concentrate in the buffy coat and the plasma just above. This is the platelet-rich plasma.

orthopedics, where it was employed to accelerate the healing of surgical wounds, damaged ligaments and tendons, and, ultimately, the treatment of OA.[3]

PRP is a biologic therapy made from a patient's own blood. "Biologic" means that a living organism made it (not a biochemist in a pharmacology lab). Biologic therapies include a spectrum of treatments, such as those made by your own body (for example, PRP, stem cells, and autologous conditioned serum) and those manufactured by bacteria or other methods. I've introduced several of these manufactured biologic therapies in earlier chapters, including the cytokine inhibitors used to treat rheumatoid arthritis, Crohn's disease, and other auto-immune conditions.

In this and future chapters, I focus on the biologic therapies that you own body produces. They are called autologous, from the Greek words *auto*, meaning "self," and *logos*, loosely translating to "relation." An autologous treatment comes from you and is given to you. Autologous biologic therapies (autobiologics), such as PRP, stem cells, and autologous conditioned serum are commonly used to treat osteoarthritis, and tendon and nerve degeneration. Because of their autobiologic nature (they are made by your own body), they are distinguished from the manufactured biologic drugs you may see advertised on television. Autobiologics are complex products that mimic the human body's own healing and repair systems.

Platelet-Rich Plasma for Osteoarthritis

Platelet-rich plasma contains hundreds of growth factors that are potentially beneficial in treating OA and other degenerative conditions. For instance, platelet-derived growth factor (PDGF) and fibroblast growth factor (FGF), which are both found in platelets, stimulate cartilage cell growth. A manufactured form of FGF has even been tested as a clinical treatment for knee OA.[4] This growth factor appeared to protect cartilage from OA damage but didn't, by itself, do much to improve pain. Another growth factor found in platelets, transforming growth factor (TGF), has been shown to relieve pain.[5] These growth factors, in combination with multiple others, have been shown to promote cartilage health and reduce the symptoms of OA.

Platelet-rich plasma also contains leukocytes, which are present in the buffy coat layer of the centrifuge tube. These leukocytes, including neutrophils and monocytes, work in concert with growth factors to stimulate healing (see Figure 6.1, page 70). Under the right conditions, this combination of growth factors and immune cells can "flip the switch" of the macrophage, creating an M2 cell and the anabolic machinery to rebuild tissues and resolve inflammation.

Several randomized trials and meta-analyses show that PRP can be more effective and longer-lasting than injections of steroids or hyaluronic acid.[6] Most of these PRP studies have been done for patients with knee OA because the knee joint is one of the most affected in the body. Research in PRP has also been done for OA of the hip, shoulder, ankle, and other joints. In these other locations, PRP has been generally but not universally effective. Results have sometimes been hindered by the types of PRP used.

Despite the important role of leukocytes in the healing cascade, there has been a surprising push in recent years to make PRP products with *reduced* concentrations of these white blood cells. These "leukocyte-reduced" PRPs have become popular, promising long-term benefits without having to experience acute inflammation or "damaging" effects of leukocytes. A few years ago, I was at a sports medicine conference where one of the speakers was making this point. He presented several publications demonstrating increased TNF, IL1, and other inflammatory cytokines in laboratory experiments that used leukocyte-rich PRP.[7] His conclusion: We should all be using leukocyte-reduced PRP to avoid the acute inflammation from PRP. Unfortunately, he ignored the steps of the healing cascade and evidence that acute inflammation can be therapeutic in proper doses. The other issue with leukocyte-reduced PRP is that the process of eliminating white blood cells also commonly reduces platelets. This means that many of the leukocyte-reduced products are also platelet-reduced. Try as they may, these products may not be able to activate the healing cascade effectively.

My concerns about low-leukocyte, low-platelet products were compounded by a 2021 publication in *The Journal of the American Medical Association*.[8] In this study, researchers randomized 144 patients with knee OA to either PRP injection or placebo (saline). When the study was completed, one of the headlines read: "PRP is no better than placebo." I immediately downloaded and sifted through the study. The patient recruitment, statistics methods, and results were solid. Strangely, I couldn't find the details of the PRP used for injection.

After a bit of digging into the publication's supplemental documents, I found that the average platelet count for "PRP" in the study was 325,000/ml. Normal blood platelet count runs from approximately 200,000/ml to 450,000/ml. In brief, the researchers studied a "platelet-rich plasma" that was not *rich* in platelets. It was a leukocyte-reduced and platelet-reduced product that could not activate a proper healing response.

This and similar studies highlight the challenge of PRP research and clinical practice. There are dozens of devices for making PRP, each producing a different concentration of platelets and leukocytes. One method may create PRP with eight times (8X) platelet concentrations. That means if the patient has 300,000 platelets/ml in their blood, their PRP contains a rich collection of 2,400,000 platelets/ml. Another type of PRP may contain platelet concentrations of 1.5 or 2X, which is not very different from the platelet concentration in the patient's blood. Varying concentrations of platelets also deliver widely divergent doses of growth factors. These details matter when it comes to healing the chronic wound of OA. Unfortunately, most blood-based regenerative therapies are lumped together and collectively called PRP regardless of their contents.

Platelet-Rich Plasma for Neuropathy

Platelet-rich plasma can also activate a healing response for nerves that have suffered from metabolic injury (diabetes), toxic injury (chemotherapy), or physical injury (carpal tunnel).

In these patients, as in patients with OA, PRP's growth factors and leukocytes can activate an immune response, transitioning microglia (the macrophages of the nervous system) to M2 cells and promoting recovery and the resolution of inflammation.[9] Two growth factors, platelet-derived growth factor (PDGF) and hepatocyte growth factor (HGF), have been shown to be critical in restoring nerve function after injury.[10] Others, such as transforming growth factor (TGF), which I discussed in Chapter 6, restore immune balance and reduce pain. In the proper concentrations, the collections of growth factors and leukocytes in PRP have been shown to improve neuropathy pain.[11]

There have been several studies of PRP for the treatment of neuropathy, especially focal nerve diseases, such as carpal tunnel syndrome. Although smaller in enrollment size, these studies have generally shown positive responses. In a meta-analysis of nine studies of PRP injections to treat carpal tunnel syndrome, PRP was found to provide better relief of pain and return of nerve function than interventions such as steroid injections.[12] PRP has also been tested to treat diffuse neuropathy from diabetes. In one study, sixty patients with diabetes, numbness, and burning pain were randomly assigned to peripheral nerve PRP injections versus standard medical management. The group that received PRP injections had significant reductions in pain. They also had improvements in nerve function with nerve conduction studies.[13] PRP augments the body's natural healing mechanisms.

Sarah's PRP Injection

After reading over the materials I gave to her, Sarah decided she wanted to proceed with a PRP injection for her knee OA pain. Before making her PRP, we first needed to optimize her chances for success. She was already following a diet rich in omega-3 fatty acids, colorful leafy greens, and olive oil. Recall the discussion of these foods and their potential benefits in Chapter 7, Fats and Plant Colors to Resolve Inflammation. Sarah also went for a brisk walk the morning of the procedure. She exercised enough to activate her immune system, but not so much that it dehydrated or exhausted her. Once she got to the clinic, I did an ultrasound exam of her knee, assessing the tendons and ligaments around her joint and checking for excess fluid (effusion) inside the joint. Sarah had no significant tendon or ligament problems but did have an effusion. This meant that I would need to drain her knee before injecting PRP but wouldn't need to do extra injections for her tendons or ligaments.

Because her OA was slightly more advanced, I also discussed with Sarah the possibility of adding a hyaluronic acid injection just before her PRP. As I discussed in Chapter 2, enzymes in OA joints break down hyaluronic acid into smaller inflammatory fragments. Although hyaluronic acid has been typically studied and used as a single intervention, it is likely more helpful in combination with PRP, where it further boosts the benefits of PRP.[14] The combination of PRP and hyaluronic acid is now common, especially in individuals more severe degenerative changes. It can be effective, even in those who experienced minimal benefits from a hyaluronic acid injection alone.

After preparing the hyaluronic acid, we were ready to make Sarah's PRP. After my assistant drew blood from her arm, I added an anticoagulant and injected the blood into a specialized centrifuge container. As Dr. Knighton had done decades earlier, we spun the blood in a centrifuge for several minutes, separating the red blood cells from the leukocytes and platelets. After removing the top layer of plasma, I attached a syringe to withdraw the platelet-rich portions of the plasma and buffy coat. This PRP had a concentration of about 6X over baseline with moderately enriched leukocytes. After draining the knee and injecting the hyaluronic acid, I then injected the PRP, watching on ultrasound as it moved freely throughout Sarah's synovial fluid, bathing the cartilage and joint surfaces.

After her injections, it took several weeks for Sarah to notice a significant difference. This is typical—almost expected. PRP takes time. Some patients even have a flare-up of pain, especially after tendon and ligament injections. It reflects the body's immune activation. After three to four weeks, Sarah began to notice improvements in her pain. She returned to playing pickleball. After about a month, she could play for extended periods and didn't need to reach for the ibuprofen as soon as she walked off the court. As Sarah's pain improved, she enjoyed her games again and time on the court with friends.

Sarah's PRP was not anti-inflammatory, nor was it a panacea that cured her OA or grew new cartilage. The platelet-rich plasma therapy she received was an immune stimulant that activated her body's natural healing responses. It contained the growth factors and leukocytes in concentrations adequate to turn on M2 macrophage activity, repair tissues, and *resolve* inflammation. For these reasons, it was a valuable tool in reducing her pain. While there are no cons of repeating this procedure other than the cost, the concept of repeat injection is still being debated.

Now that you know about PRP, its immune effects, and its potential uses, it's time to explore one of the most controversial regenerative therapies: stem cells. You'll learn how the stem cells used to treat OA and neuropathy differ from embryonic stem cells and how they, like platelet-rich plasma, also modify immune function.

Takeaways

1. PRP was first employed in the management of nonhealing wounds before it was used to treat osteoarthritis.
2. PRP is made from a patient's own blood and contains variable concentrations of platelets, growth factors, and leukocytes.
3. With the right dose, PRP activates the natural healing cascade and can decrease pain from osteoarthritis and neuropathy.

Chapter 12

Are "Stem Cells" Really Stem Cells?

As Marcus sought options for his sciatica pain after surgery, he found an advertisement for a stem cell treatment. He printed the promotion and brought it to his clinic visit with me. The ad promised amniotic stem cells that would restore nerves, regrow cartilage, reverse Parkinson's disease, and cure many other ailments. Marcus was excited to see this. He wondered, could stem cells also stop his pain and repair his sciatic nerve? A short answer to his questions wasn't easy. To fully grasp the potential (and the limitations) of stem cells, we must visit the 1960s and the pioneering work of Dr. Arnold Caplan.

The Discovery of Adult Stem Cells

In the 1960s, Dr. Caplan completed his PhD at The Johns Hopkins University School of Medicine, where his studies focused on understanding mitochondrial function. After receiving his degree, he began working on a new project to unravel the causes of several muscle and cartilage defects. To decipher these developmental defects, Caplan had to first know how tissues, such as cartilage, muscle, bone, and adipose (fat), grew from a single type of stem cell. He began studying chick embryos, acquiring a deep knowledge of how their cells matured and developed.

In 1969, Dr. Caplan was recruited to Case Western Reserve University in Cleveland to teach developmental biology and continue his research. In his laboratory experiments, he found that a particular type of chick embryo stem cell could develop into cartilage, muscle, bone, or adipose tissue depending on the growth factors and conditions present. The stem cells he studied made "middle" connective tissues that unite outer tissues (skin) and inner tissues (intestines, lungs, etc.) and bind chick embryos (and humans) together. These middle tissues—such as cartilage, muscle, bone, and adipose—give people strength, motion, and function. He named the stem cells that created these tissues "mesenchymal" (meh-ZEN-kih-mul from the Greek *meso*, meaning "middle" and *chyme* for bodily tissue/fluid.

One of Dr. Caplan's important early discoveries was that mesenchymal stem cells (MSCs) were not only present in chick embryos but also in human adult tissues, such as bone marrow. It was a "eureka" moment. If MSCs were present in all adults and MSCs naturally develop into tissues like cartilage, could an individual donate bone marrow to regenerate their own cartilage? Using bone marrow would not only give patients a near-endless supply of stem cells, but it would also eliminate ethical concerns about embryonic cells or fetal tissues. An individual could obtain all the stem cells they needed from their own bodies.

Dr. Caplan began honing methods for growing adult stem cells and turning them into chondrocytes to produce new cartilage. The first step was to separate the stem cells from the other bone marrow cells. This separation was important because MSCs comprise only 0.001–0.01 percent of the bone marrow cells. Before growing stem cells, he needed to remove 99.99 percent of the other (unwanted) cells.

Dr. Caplan found out that MSCs had a unique property that helped him separate the cells—they're sticky. The rest of the bone marrow makes blood cells built to flow freely in arteries and veins. MSCs are different. As connective tissue cells, they are built to adhere to surfaces. MSCs not only stick to other tissues in the body, but also to the bottom of a cell culture dish. Caplan found that if he added bone marrow to culture dishes and waited, the MSCs would adhere, and he could simply rinse off the other cells. Once he had a plate with a few MSCs stuck to the bottom, he could add nutrients to multiply the MSCs into the millions. This multiplication step, called culturing, took several weeks to produce enough cells for use. Caplan also discovered that if he added specific growth factors, he could coax the MSCs into becoming chondrocytes, producers of new cartilage (Figure 12.1). In 1991, he published his techniques for growing cartilage from adult bone marrow cells. His potential cure for osteoarthritis set the regenerative medicine world on fire.[1]

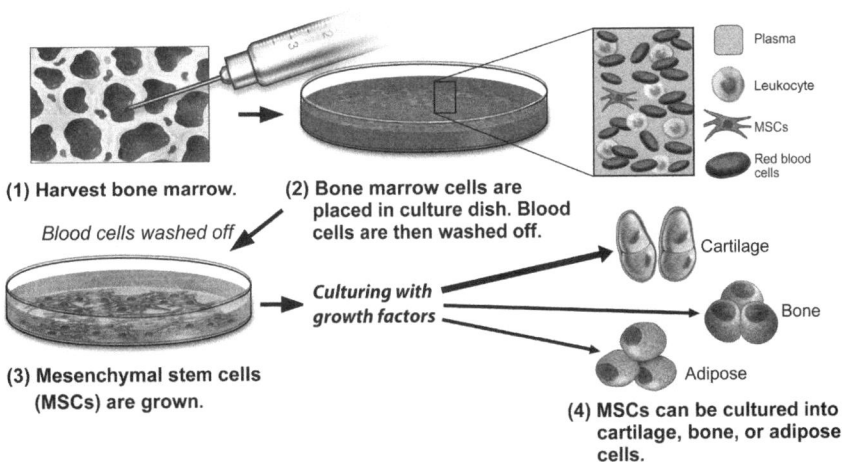

(1) Harvest bone marrow.

(2) Bone marrow cells are placed in culture dish. Blood cells are then washed off.

Blood cells washed off

(3) Mesenchymal stem cells (MSCs) are grown.

Culturing with growth factors

(4) MSCs can be cultured into cartilage, bone, or adipose cells.

Plasma

Leukocyte

MSCs

Red blood cells

Cartilage

Bone

Adipose

Figure 12.1. Mesenchymal stem cells (MSCs): (1) Bone marrow is harvested with a needle. (2) The marrow cells are placed in a culture dish. MSCs adhere to the dish, and the other cells are rinsed away. (3) The MSCs are grown for several weeks until enough cells are available for use. (4) Growth factors can be added to culture the cells into cartilage, bone, or adipose tissue.

The Race to Grow New Cartilage

After Dr. Caplan's publication, the race was on to regenerate cartilage. The early results were exciting. In one experiment, the effects of MSCs were tested in goats. Goats, like humans, are prone to knee OA after injuries to the meniscus or ligaments. The scientists worked with 24 goats who had both meniscus and ligament tears and were rapidly developing OA. Under anesthesia, their bone marrow was extracted and placed in a culture dish. After washing off the nonsticky marrow cells, researchers grew the MSCs for several weeks. They then added a fluorescent dye to the MSCs so the location of the cells could be tracked over time. Two thirds of the goat knees were injected with 10 million glowing MSCs. The other damaged joints were injected with hyaluronic acid (HA), the large lubricant molecules I introduced in Chapter 1, Joint Anatomy and the Myth of "Wear and Tear." After several months, the goat knees were examined under a microscope. The joints that received MSCs had the fluorescent cells still glowing in their joints. They also had less OA and meniscus damage. The MSCs appeared to restore meniscus health and protect the joints from developing OA.[2]

Enthusiasm about MSCs further swelled after the publication about a patient with knee OA who was successfully treated with these cells.[3] The researchers used Dr. Caplan's technique of harvesting bone marrow and growing the MSCs in a culture dish until they had several million MSCs. These stem cells, along with PRP from the patient's blood, were then injected into his arthritic knee. His pain significantly improved. The authors also compared several MRI images before and six months after the injection and described improvements in cartilage thickness.

Following these positive results, several controlled studies were completed to more rigorously test the effects of MSCs in individuals with knee OA. In 2015, Spanish researchers reported the results of thirty patients who were randomly assigned to receive injections of either MSCs or hyaluronic acid for their knee OA.[4] All the participants also had knee MRIs performed before and twelve months after the injection. To accurately assess any cartilage changes, the researchers used a specialized MRI tool. An MRI normally takes images at different angles through the joint. When a physician or surgeon reviews these "slices" as part of a clinical assessment, they are "flipping" through multiple images, right to left, front to back. With this process, the MRI viewer assembles a complete picture of the joint in their mind. This process, although effective for clinical care, isn't accurate enough for research purposes. Another process to compare before and after MRIs is to line up and directly compare individual slices. This technique also has challenges. Slice #7–9 on one MRI scan rarely lines up with slice #7–9 on another. To overcome these measurement challenges, the Spanish researchers employed an MRI tool that systematically evaluated multiple areas of cartilage and calculated an overall cartilage "index." In this manner, the scientists could determine if the cartilage changed over time. This tool, although accurate in assessing changes in cartilage health, wasn't designed to determine regrowth. They would be able to tell if cartilage improved in quality but not if new cartilage was being made. When the researchers compared the before and after MRIs, they found that the individuals who received MSCs had significantly better cartilage quality than those who received hyaluronic acid.

Irrational Exuberance for Stem Cell–Grown Cartilage?

Despite the enthusiasm generated from early stem cell publications, there were still knowledge gaps. Goats aren't humans. It's hard to judge cartilage regrowth by comparing individual slices from MRIs. Improvements in cartilage health aren't the same as growing new cartilage. MSCs appeared to offer benefits, but how they did so was unclear.

Scientists began to question the concept that the pain relief from stem cells was due to growing new cartilage. That challenge grew louder in 2019 with the publication of a study from Vienna, Austria.[5] In this research, scientists started with the standard technique of growing MSCs in a culture dish from bone marrow. The researchers then chemically labeled the MSCs, allowing them to track the cells for months. The labeled MSCs were injected into the arthritic joints of laboratory animals and were soon found embedded in areas of damaged cartilage. The researchers then waited. And waited. What they observed over time was unexpected. The stem cells died off. Most were gone after a couple of months. Curiously, as the stem cells were dying, the cartilage health was improving. The healing response seemed disconnected from stem cell survival.

The death of MSCs after injection was a surprise to many physicians and surgeons, but probably not to a research group from Seoul, South Korea. These researchers had already done a unique study of MSCs for patients with knee OA. Rather than inject the MSCs into the knee joint with a needle, they surgically applied the cells directly to the areas of cartilage damage. Then, they gave the patients braces and strict instructions not to put any weight on the knee for two weeks. The researchers wanted to ensure the MSCs weren't displaced from their implant location. In the subsequent weeks, the patients were slowly allowed to return to activities. The clinical results were impressive. Ninety-four percent of the patients experienced significant improvements in both pain and function. Approximately a year after their stem cell implant, the study participants had additional surgery to directly visualize the surface of their knee and record the extent of cartilage regrowth. Shockingly, more than 75 percent of the patients still had significant damage. The implanted stem cells reduced pain without growing new cartilage.[6]

Researchers from Chile saw comparable results in their study of patients with moderate knee OA. Participants underwent MRI scans and were randomly assigned to receive injections of either stem cells or hyaluronic acid (HA) into their knees.[7] Those who received stem cells experienced greater pain relief at one year than those who received HA. The researchers repeated the MRIs at 6 and 12 months. Like the Spanish investigators, they used an MRI measurement tool to systematically assess multiple areas of cartilage for thickness and health. Despite the greater pain relief in those who received MSCs, there was no significant difference between the cartilage of those who received stem cells and those who received HA. In 2020, researchers published a meta-analysis of stem cell studies and came to the same conclusion. Stem cells may produce pain relief, but it isn't from cartilage regrowth.[8]

The FDA Clamps Down on Stem Cells in the US

If you've had a friend or relative who has had a stem cell procedure, they may have described to you an injection that was done right after cells were collected. This represents a significant change from the original stem cell techniques developed by Dr. Caplan. This change came about largely because of safety concerns by the Federal Drug Administration (FDA). The process of culturing stem cells not only takes time but also requires strict adherence to sterile technique. Unless they are kept in a meticulous laboratory, cells can become contaminated with bacteria, fungi, or viruses, and the complications can be severe. In the US, there have been reports of infections, paralysis, and even death with cultured stem cells.[9] These concerns prompted the FDA to tighten regulations in 2021, requiring any individual or company growing these cells to undergo an approval process and rigorous quality testing. These more stringent standards shut down nearly all the individual clinics and companies culturing stem cells.

Stem cell procedures now commonly start with collecting cells from a source such as bone marrow. At this point, the process diverges from Dr. Caplan's method. Rather than growing cells for weeks in culture dishes, an anticoagulant is added and the bone marrow cells are put into a centrifuge. After spinning at high speeds, the cells, like blood components, separate by weight. Heavy cells on the bottom, light cells on the top.

MSCs have a weight similar to leukocytes and, therefore, settle out near the "buffy coat" in a centrifuge, as platelets in PRP do. The buffy coat layer (containing MSCs and leukocytes) is siphoned off and immediately injected (Figure 12.2). This material, which many still call "stem cells," is more appropriately referred to as a "bone marrow concentrate." It contains leukocytes and bone marrow cells with a few MSCs mixed in (recall that MSCs make up only about 0.001–0.01 percent of bone marrow cells).

You may have also heard of stem cells from adipose (fat) tissue. In this process, small amounts of adipose are removed from the patient, usually from the abdomen and flank, with a liposuction-type device. There are more MSCs in adipose tissue than in bone marrow, but still not many. MSCs comprise about 1 percent of the cells collected with this liposuction process. After the adipose tissue is collected, the larger fat cells must be removed. There are different ways of doing this. Some processes involve mechanically breaking up the fat particles by shaking them with metal beads and filtering them. Others use a centrifuge to separate the cells by weight, similar to bone marrow

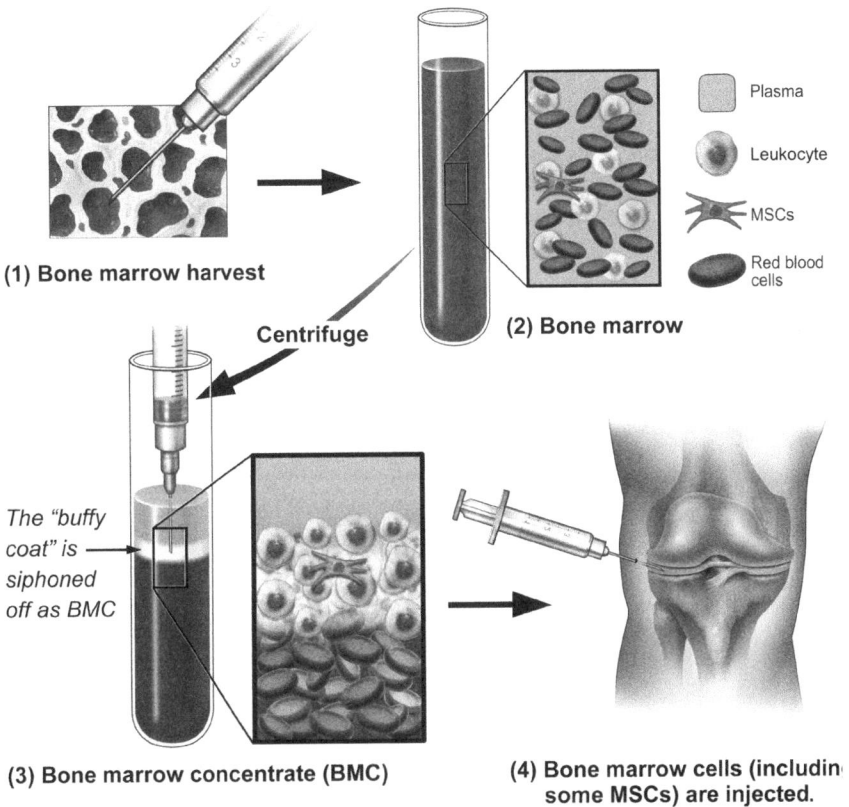

Figure 12.2. Bone marrow concentrate: Bone marrow is harvested, anticoagulated, and centrifuged. The "buffy coat" and surrounding cells are siphoned off. The bone marrow concentrate is still commonly referred to as a "stem cell" procedure.

concentrate or PRP. Once the larger cells are removed, the rest of the adipose cells and MSCs are immediately injected. There is no growing or culturing of cells. There are fewer risks—and fewer MSCs. Nonetheless, the phrase "stem cell therapy" continues to live on, regardless of the concentration of MSCs present or the use of culturing techniques.

Patients and physicians have wondered if bone marrow or adipose cell concentrates are as effective as traditionally grown MSCs for treating osteoarthritis and other degenerative conditions. A 2021 meta-analysis of stem cell procedures (both culture-grown MSCs and cell concentrates) explored this question. The investigators concluded that while both techniques may be helpful for pain, cultured cells may be slightly more effective.[10] However, a more recent clinical trial contradicted these findings. The investigators directly compared multiple interventions, including bone marrow concentrate, adipose concentrate, and culture-grown stem cells to treating knee OA. There was no difference in pain relief between the procedures and no advantage of using cultured MSCs.[11]

In 2020, another head-to-head comparison was completed, this time between bone marrow concentrate and PRP for patients with knee OA. When the investigators evaluated the patients after a year, they found that both interventions reduced pain equally. There was no advantage of using MSCs rather than PRP.[12] This is good news for anyone seeking a biologic therapy for their OA pain. PRP may provide the same benefits as a more painful (and more costly) bone marrow procedure.

Amniotic, Placental, and Umbilical Stem Cells

So far, I've presented the details about bone marrow and adipose stem cells. What about Marcus's initial questions regarding amniotic stem cells? Like bone marrow and adipose tissue, birth tissues, such as amniotic fluid, placenta, and umbilical cord, contain MSCs in varying concentrations. These tissues, usually discarded after birth, fall under the category of "allogenic" products. *Allo* is derived from the Greek for "other," signifying that the cell donor and recipient are different people.

Allogenic treatments may have some advantages as people age, providing "youthful" cells and growth factors. Donated tissues also carry additional risks of infection or contamination. There are several active research studies of amniotic tissue products for the treatment of OA pain with promising early results.[13] But at the time of Marcus's question (and the writing of this chapter), there is no FDA-approved amniotic, placental, or umbilical tissue product approved for use in the US for arthritis. The advertisement that Marcus saw was for a stem cell product that is no longer available and was possibly of unclear safety. Regenerative therapies remain the Wild West of medicine.

If you or a loved one are seeking a stem cell therapy option, all of these various treatments might be a bit confusing. Fortunately, there is a simple question you can ask to help guide you: "Is the stem cell (MSC) treatment being used as part of the practice of medicine?" If you're offered a free steak dinner to listen to a sales pitch about the latest "miracle" stem cell product, it is no longer the practice of medicine. If you're given a menu of stem cell options and asked to check off the ones you'd like to receive, it's no longer the practice of medicine. If you're told that 100 percent of patients respond to a treatment, it's not true. If you're told that an amniotic or placental product is sterilized for safety and contains "live stem cells," it's not true. Any sterilization process will also kill any living cells. These are sales pitches with the primary goal of making money, not helping you.

There are several wonderful examples of how regenerative medicine can be practiced ethically, appropriately, and in a patient-centered manner. The Mayo Clinic in Jacksonville, Florida, is one such program. Clinicians and scientists in their regenerative medicine program offer autobiologic therapies such as PRP and MSCs and routinely include counseling before any intervention. The Mayo Clinic doctors have worked hard to make sure the patients understand the potential benefits and limitations of these therapies. Many other individual physician's and surgeon's practices also offer PRP and MSC treatments conscientiously and ethically. Just steer clear of free steak dinners, claims of miracle cures, and deals that sound too good to be true.

I had a similar discussion of the pros and cons of MSCs with Marcus. After this conversation, he decided to hold off. He was feeling progressive improvements in pain and function with his physical therapy and exercise program. He noted he would reconsider regenerative therapies later if needed.

A Name Change for MSCs

As his research progressed, Dr. Caplan became increasingly aware of the disconnect between what stem cells do in a culture dish and what they do inside people's bodies. In 2010, he penned an editorial imploring scientists and clinicians to stop using the term "mesenchymal stem cells."[14] He urged changing the name of MSCs from "mesenchymal stem cells" to "medicinal signaling cells." This new name reflected their function of improving the health of the cells around them, not by growing new tissues. His research conclusions were undeniable. MSCs were medicinal.

This editorial was a remarkable moment in science. The father of "mesenchymal stem cells" voluntarily retracted the name he bestowed upon these cells thirty years earlier. With this name change of MSCs to "medicinal signaling cells," Dr. Caplan simultaneously respected history and turned the page on "stem cells." The acronym "MSC" remained a linguistic link to decades of past research, and "medicinal" now reflected the function of these cells. Like PRP, MSCs activate the immune system. Precisely how MSCs provide these medicinal benefits and pain relief is the topic of the next chapter.

Takeaways

1. Dr. Arnold Caplan first cultured stem cells (MSCs) from adult bone marrow with hopes of regrowing cartilage in arthritic joints.
2. In the United States, restrictions on culturing stem cells were tightened by the FDA in 2021. This increased regulation led to the common use of bone marrow and adipose cell concentrates.
3. MSCs are now commonly referred to as medicinal signaling cells, reflecting their function and the release of medicinal factors.

Chapter 13

MSCs: Immune System Regulators

In the last chapter, I discussed how Dr. Arnold Caplan taught the medical community that medicinal signaling cells (MSCs) provide pain relief through the factors they release, not the tissues they grow. Thanks to scientists such as Dr. Ru-Rong Ji at Duke Anesthesiology's Center for Translational Pain Medicine in Durham, physicians now know what some of those factors are and how they work. Dr. Ji has spent decades studying the response of spinal cord immune cells to nerve injury and how this response determines whether pain resolves or becomes chronic. His insights and research have also illuminated how MSCs reduce pain.

The Effect of MSCs on Nerve Pain

Dr. Ji knew MSCs had medicinal effects and knew the "medicines" they secreted were still not clearly understood. He designed a series of experiments to understand their mechanisms. Like Dr. Caplan, Ji started with bone marrow cells to generate his MSCs. His team put mice under anesthesia, harvested the marrow, and added it to culture dishes in a controlled laboratory environment. After the MSC adhered to the dish, and he rinsed away the rest of the marrow cells, nutrients were added and the cells were grown for several weeks. He also attached a fluorescent dye to the cells, so they would glow when viewed under specialized microscopes in order to track the cells after injection.

At this point in the experiment, Dr. Ji's work diverged from Dr. Caplan's. Rather than put the MSCs into knees or other arthritic joints, he chose to inject the cells into the spinal fluid of mice with nerve injuries.[1] This difference was an essential step in understanding how MSCs relieved pain. If the MSCs grew new cartilage or other mesenchymal tissues, such as bone or muscle, it would have been disastrous around the spine. The injected mice would experience permanent spinal cord damage. But Dr. Ji knew the science and was confident this wouldn't happen. He knew MSCs worked by secreting various factors. He just didn't know yet what all those factors were.

The mice he chose to treat were affected by a nerve injury similar to sciatica in people. Like Marcus, who limped with the pain of his disc herniation, the mice avoided placing pressure on the affected limbs. They also became quite sensitive to touch. This sensitivity was tested with a thin filament. Normally, touching the paw of a mouse with this filament was barely noticed by the animal. But, with nerve pain, even the slightest touch could be painful. Pain relief in the mice was measured by decreased sensitivity to touch and improvements in motion. In other words, their skin became less sensitive, and they walked better. In addition to improvements in pain, Dr. Ji's team also measured the proteins and growth factors that the MSCs produced, trying to gain insight into how these cells worked.

Within days of the MSC injection, the skin sensitivity and movement of the mice improved. When Dr. Ji's team examined the animals' nerves and spinal cords with a microscope, they saw MSCs sitting on the surface of these structures. With the use of special stains, the team also noted reduced spinal cord inflammation. Ji followed the changes over time. The injected

MSCs lived for several weeks and then died off. As expected, no cartilage or bone was produced. Even though the MSCs weren't living long, they were reducing pain and resolving inflammation in the spine.

The team then measured the proteins and growth factors secreted by the MSCs. They found a spike in transforming growth factor (TGF), the growth factor introduced in Chapter 6, Igniting the Immune System to Heal. In joints with osteoarthritis, TGF helps re-establish immune cell balance and resolve chronic inflammation. In nerves, TGF has a similar effect. Dr. Ji knew it was important to find out if this spike in TGF was *driving* pain relief or just acting as a bystander. To do so, he employed an antibody to TGF. When injected, the antibody shuts down the effects of TGF without affecting other MSC functions. If TGF were driving the effect, pain would return with the antibody. If TGF were a bystander, the antibody would have no effect. His team injected the TGF antibody and retested paw sensitivity to the filaments. The mice nerve pain returned. The answer was clear. The MSCs were making TGF, and this growth factor produced pain relief.

Neural MSCs for Spinal Cord Injury?

Around the same time that Dr. Ji was studying the effects of MSCs to reduce nerve injury pain, the medical community was also becoming very interested in MSCs to treat spinal cord injury. Scientists discovered that by using special growth factors, they could culture MSCs into neuronlike cells. Regular MSCs didn't live for more than a few weeks around the spine. Might "neural" MSCs fare better? Could these neuronlike cells regrow damaged parts of the spinal cord and reverse the devastating effects of this injury?

Neural MSCs were tested in several different laboratories by researchers studying spinal cord injury, including a team from

South Korea. At this lab, researchers labeled neural MSCs with fluorescent dyes and injected them directly into the injured spinal cords of rats. After four weeks, the scientists examined the spinal cords under a microscope. The MSCs were seen glowing with life at the injection site. Even more encouraging, many of them were looking and behaving like neurons. The research team was thrilled at the possibility of a cell treatment for spinal cord repair. The researchers waited another four weeks and rechecked the spinal cords. This time, the MSCs were nowhere to be found. They had died off, just like regular MSCs did. Although it was possible to grow MSCs into neuronlike cells, this process did not help their survival in the spinal cord.[2] Despite their brief lives, the cells still acted in a "medicinal" fashion. When the researchers measured nerve conduction velocities in the damaged areas, they were faster. When they tested the animals' walk, they regained some ability to move. The neural MSCs didn't live for long, but they improved the function of the nerves around them.

MSCs Stimulate the Immune System

When injected around peripheral nerves or the spine, MSCs release TGF and other medicinal factors that improve pain. What if these cells were given intravenously, into a vein far away from the nerve injury? Would they still improve pain? At the Cleveland Clinic, Dr. Jianguo Cheng, designed experiments to answer this question. Cheng's team assessed the effects of different MSC injections in rats with nerve injury pain. They began by culturing MSCs from bone marrow and adipose cells and then added fluorescent labels to those cells. They then injected the MSCs into the spinal fluid of some rats and the veins of others.[3]

The team observed and tested the animals for several weeks after injection. Pain was assessed by measuring the sensitivity of the rats' paws to thin filaments and warm temperatures. There was no difference between the effects of MSCs made from bone marrow and those made from adipose cells. Both of these types of cells reduced paw sensitivity. This was unsurprising since the cells were grown with similar techniques. The surprise was that the animals who received the intravenous MSCs did as well as those who had MSCs in the spinal fluid. Did the intravenous MSCs migrate to the spine, or was there some other mechanism involved?

Dr. Cheng and colleagues examined the spinal cords of the animals a few weeks after injection. Those who received MSCs in their spinal fluid still had these cells glowing on the surface of the spinal cord, releasing TGF and other pain-relieving factors. The research team then examined the spinal cords of the rats who received the intravenous MSCs (who also experienced improvements in their pain). There were no visible MSCs on or around the spine. The rats had improved pain without the MSCs ever reaching their nerve targets. Something else was driving pain relief besides the local release of "medicines."

The answer to the mystery of pain relief after intravenous cell injection came from scientific teams from the US, UK, Netherlands, China, and Japan.[4] These researchers found that intravenous MSCs in rats and mice were consumed by macrophages soon after injection. Although that process destroyed the MSCs, it flipped the switch on the animals' macrophages, transitioning the macrophages to M2 cells. As they do after an injury, these M2 macrophages became mini-factories, pumping out pain-relieving growth factors, such as TGF, inflammation-resolving cytokines, such as IL-10, and SPMs, such as resolvins and protectins (Figure 12.1 on page 143). The MSCs were stimulating the immune system.

To confirm that macrophages, and not other immune cells, were responsible for pain relief, the researchers then ran two

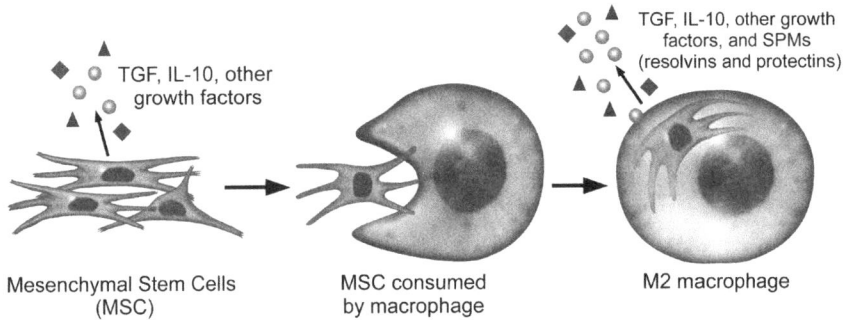

Figure 13.1. Pain relief from MSCs: MSCs work by (1) secreting TGF and and other growth factors and (2) activating M2 macrophages that produce additional growth factors and SPMs such as resolvins and protectins.

additional sets of experiments. First, they chemically eliminated the macrophages from the laboratory animals and reinjected MSCs. With the macrophages gone, no M2 cells could be created. The animals' pain relief from the MSCs was significantly reduced.

In a second experiment, they treated nerve-injured rats with MSCs and confirmed pain relief. They then removed their macrophages and injected them into animals with the same nerve injury (who hadn't been treated with MSCs). The recipient rats experienced pain relief.[5] By transferring the macrophages, they transferred the pain relief. The results were unequivocal. More critical than releasing their own growth factors, the MSCs relieved the pain by flipping the immune switch and creating M2 cells (Figure 13.1).

Can MSCs Resolve a Difficult Pain Condition?

The ability of MSCs to flip the immune switch and create M2 cells caught the attention of Dr. Cheng. As a pain management specialist, he treated patients with various nerve-pain conditions, including a difficult condition called complex regional pain syndrome (CRPS). Patients with CRPS experience severe pain, swelling, and even temperature changes in the affected area. The pain can be triggered by the slightest touch—a bedsheet brushing against the foot or a shirt sleeve touching the arm. CRPS-like disorders have been described for centuries, but a US Army neurologist, Dr. Silas Weir Mitchell, offered the first complete descriptions in 1864. He treated injured American Civil War soldiers, noting that some had lingering nerve pain, even after the resolution of the wound. Mitchell wrote about CRPS (that he called at the time "causalgia"), describing it as "the most terrible of all the tortures which a nerve wound may inflict."[6]

Despite centuries of research to understand CRPS, this nerve-pain syndrome has continued to elude effective treatments. Pain specialists use medications, nerve injections, surgeries, and even electrical stimulation. Sometimes the interventions work. Sometimes they don't. CRPS can also be diagnostically confusing. The redness, warmth, and swelling of a foot or a hand appears inflammatory and sometimes like an infection. Frequently, the patients are treated (unsuccessfully) with antibiotics. The cause is not an infection. The swelling, temperature changes, and pain are due to a nerve injury that causes the immune system to go haywire.

The details of the immune dysfunction with CRPS have become increasingly clear through recent research by Dr. David Clark and his colleagues at Stanford University.[7] Their team has been studying the serum of patients with CRPS, trying to understand the immune factors that drive the pain and inflammation of this condition. Serum is what remains of blood when the cells are allowed to clot and are then removed (usually with the help of a centrifuge). The resulting clear yellow fluid contains the proteins, cytokines, growth factors, and antibodies from the blood. Serum contains the products of immune cells without the cells themselves.

Dr. Clark and his colleagues performed multiple experiments to determine if the serum of patients with CRPS could "transmit" pain. In one set of experiments, they injected serum from patients with CRPS and serum from healthy donors (without CRPS) into mice with fractures, a common type of injury leading to CRPS. As expected, healthy donor serum had no effect. When CRPS patient serum was injected into the same mice, it significantly worsened their pain. The immune imbalance of the CRPS patient serum could be transferred to recreate pain.

Dr. Cheng began to connect these dots. If an immune imbalance causes the pain of CRPS, and MSCs create M2 macrophages that re-establish immune balance, could MSCs be used to treat CRPS? Cheng designed a study to find out. He has received funding from the National Institutes of Health to study MSCs to see if they can reverse CRPS, this "most terrible of tortures." His research protocol is undergoing initial (and extensive) safety testing with the institute and the FDA. If all goes as planned, he will begin enrolling patients in the study in the next few years. Optimism is high in the pain management community that he may have an effective treatment for CRPS that strikes at the heart of this disease—immune dysfunction. His research study may finally provide an answer to this elusive pain condition.

MSCs Without the Cells?

Scientists now know that MSCs don't grow new nerves or cartilage. They release local "medicines" and stimulate the body's healing responses, such as M2 macrophages. This immune response releases growth factors and inflammation-resolving cytokines and lipids. This process also releases another critical component—exosomes. In Chapter 8, Exercise, Inflammation, and Joint Healing, I discussed how exosomes from exercise promote nerve, cartilage, and muscle recovery. Exosomes are also produced by the MSCs and the M2 macrophages they create and are potent tools for healing that have been tested to treat OA.

An Italian research group performed a direct comparison between MSCs and exosomes. They studied these two therapies in rats with rapidly progressive osteoarthritis. The team began by culturing MSCs using standard techniques. They then made a significant change. Typically, when MSCs are prepared for injection, the culture fluid that bathes the cells is thrown out. In contrast, these researchers saved the culture fluid. This fluid doesn't have MSCs but contains all the proteins and exosomes the MSCs had secreted. The scientists took the culture fluid, removed the parts they didn't need, and concentrated the exosomes.

As the animals developed arthritis, they were divided into two groups. One group had their knees injected with 500,000 cultured MSCs. The other group was injected with the exosomes isolated from the culture fluid. The researchers observed the rats for three weeks and then retested their pain by assessing their sensitivity to knee pressure. Both groups of rats had significant improvements in pain. When they analyzed the cartilage under a microscope, both groups were also protected from developing severe OA.

The researchers then tested the immune cells in the joints. In both the group of rats that received MSCs and those that received exosomes, the macrophages transitioned to M2 cells. The exosomes were as effective as the MSCs in flipping the immune switch to improve their pain and protect their cartilage.[8] It turns out that the animals didn't need the MSCs at all—only the exosomes.

Medicinal Cells and Lessons Learned

Drs. Caplan, Ji, Cheng, and others have taught valuable lessons regarding MSCs and how they work. Dr. Caplan showed the importance of these cells and how to grow them from bone marrow. He gave us laboratory techniques to culture MSCs into cartilage cells—and the hope of curing osteoarthritis. As his research progressed, he realized that MSCs in the body don't regrow cartilage, nerves, or other tissues. Instead MSCs act in a "medicinal" manner," affecting the immune cells around them. Dr. Ji taught us that MSCs release growth factors such as TGF that can improve the pain of nerve injury and orthopedic conditions. Now, Dr. Cheng is exploring the ability of MSCs to provide pain relief for patients with CRPS, a nerve-pain condition that has escaped effective treatments for centuries.

Another critical lesson is that exosomes may be as effective as MSCs in producing pain relief and slowing the development of OA. These immune vesicles are released from multiple cell types, including MSCs and macrophages, and have the ability, if the conditions are right, to improve the health and function of the cells around them. The immune mechanisms and the process of manufacturing the most effective exosomes to treat OA and neuropathy pain are finally being understood. Some of this understanding is through research the team I work with has done on a biologic therapy called autologous conditioned serum—the topic of the next chapter.

Takeaways

1. The pain relief from MSCs is partly due to TGF and inflammation-resolving cytokines.
2. MSCs have a limited lifespan after injection. They provide benefits by activating inflammation-resolving M2 macrophage cells.
3. The exosomes secreted by M2 macrophages and MSCs may be as effective as the MSCs themselves in alleviating osteoarthritis and neuropathy pain.

Chapter 14

Autologous Conditioned Serum: A Professional and Personal Journey

In previous chapters, I presented the importance of immune stimulation, growth factors, and inflammation-resolving cytokines in treating osteoarthritis (OA) and neuropathy. Platelet-rich plasma (PRP) releases growth factors and stimulates the immune system. Mesenchymal stem cells (MSCs), or medicinal signaling cells, turn on the healing mechanisms of the M2 macrophage. This chapter will discuss a third regenerative therapy called autologous conditioned serum (ACS). ACS differs significantly from PRP. ACS also doesn't require harvesting bone marrow or adipose cells like MSCs do. To appreciate how ACS works, we need to look back a few decades, specifically to the 1980s and the contributions of a German orthopedic surgeon, Dr. Peter Wehling.

The Birth of ACS

In the 1980s, Dr. Wehling had finished medical school and was training in orthopedic surgery in Düsseldorf, Germany. He was skilled with his hands and enjoyed the long days in the operating room. But as his orthopedic residency progressed, he became increasingly puzzled by a disconnect he saw in patients undergoing spine surgery. That disconnect was between the severity of the spinal nerve compression and the severity of sciatica pain. The traditional medical assumption was that more compression led to more pain. Dr. Wehling realized there was little correlation between the two. Something else was driving the pain. It was inflammation. Surgery reduced the pressure on the nerves but didn't directly reduce the inflammation. Corticosteroids effectively treated the inflammation, but, often the benefits were only temporary. He was determined to find a better solution for his patients.

Dr. Wehling discussed this with colleagues. He also began reaching out to scientists around the globe, hoping to study this question in greater depth. It became rapidly evident where he needed to go—the University of Pittsburgh with the internationally known researcher, Dr. Chris Evans. Dr. Evans is an expert in inflammation and pain, and, at the time, he was studying the newly discovered cytokine proteins that controlled the immune system. Wehling was offered and accepted a fellowship position to begin work in Evan's laboratory immediately after finishing his orthopedic residency.

Drs. Wehling and Evans quickly got to work. To find an effective and long-lasting treatment for sciatica, they first needed to understand what caused the pain of disc herniation and other nerve compressions. They designed a set of experiments in rats with disc herniations and found that inflammatory cytokines, such as IL-1, were the culprits. They then blocked this cytokine with IL-1Ra (discussed in Chapter 2, How to Damage Cartilage) and observed that doing so effectively reduced both inflammation and pain.[1] The scientific conclusions were clear: The pain of sciatica was driven by cytokines, and the pain could be reversed without steroids. Their discoveries became the foundation for the later development of ACS.

After completing his research fellowship in Pittsburgh, Dr. Wehling returned to Düsseldorf, where he became an orthopedic spine surgeon. He used his surgical skills to treat patients with various spine disorders, such as disc herniations or narrowing around spinal nerves (see the discussion of spinal stenosis on page 54 in Chapter 5, Current Nerve Treatments). He was conscientious when offering surgery to patients, knowing that he was treating compression but not always the inflammation that caused pain.

He realized it was time for a new approach. He decided to establish a company to bring his Pittsburgh research discoveries to patients. Dr. Julio Reinecke, a German PhD scientist and expert in cellular biology, joined, and they began testing methods to treat the pain caused by cytokines. They knew IL-1Ra was a powerful tool and explored multiple techniques to enhance this inflammation resolver. Some methods were successful but overly complex for use in the clinic. The team still needed to find a reliable and safe solution for patients.

Drs. Wehling, Reinecke, Evans, and their colleagues then returned to the body's natural immune response to injury. After months of trial and error, they discovered that if blood were allowed to clot under mildly stressful incubator conditions, immune cells pumped out IL-1Ra, TGF, IL-10, and other pain-relieving factors.[2] The most significant effect they observed was with IL-1Ra, which multiplied up to a 100✕ baseline. The immune cells, as they do in the body, were sensing the acute inflammatory stress and responding to resolve the inflammation. Later, it was determined that this effect was from the M2 macrophage, but their research preceded this discovery. The team found a way to naturally produce inflammation-resolving cytokines to treat the nerve pain that Wehling and Evans had seen in the laboratory, and Wehling saw in his patients. They standardized the process, added strict sterility protocols, and named it autologous conditioned serum (ACS) (Figure 14.1 on page 170).

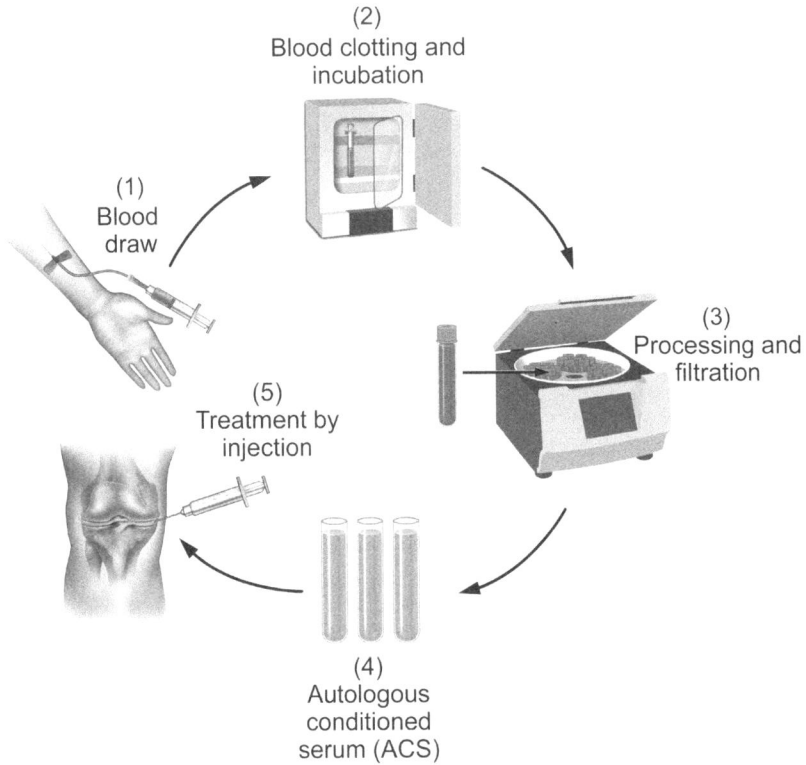

Figure 14.1. Autologous conditioned serum (ACS): ACS begins when blood is allowed to clot under strict incubation conditions. After extended clotting, the blood is centrifuged to remove the cells. The remaining serum with inflammation-resolving cytokines and other factors is called ACS.

ACS in the Clinic

Once the product and procedure was standardized, Dr. Wehling began studying the effects of ACS on patients in the clinic. Because he is a spine surgeon, many of the individuals he evaluated were suffering from sciatica despite steroid injections, physical therapy, and, sometimes, surgery. With ACS, he saw symptoms improve in many who previously had intractable pain. Speaking years later, he told me, "After I saw the results of ACS in the first twenty patients, I knew we had something special." In 1998, Wehling, Reinecke, and other colleagues published their results comparing ACS to corticosteroid injections. They found that those who received ACS experienced better and more prolonged pain relief.[3] Similar results were also observed in a later study of ACS for sciatica, where patients continued to improve, even at six months.[4]

The use of ACS quickly expanded to treating osteoarthritis with equal success. A large, blinded, randomized trial of nearly four hundred participants with knee OA revealed superior outcomes of ACS over hyaluronic acid or placebo injections. This study was also unique in its length. The standard timeframe to assess an intervention for arthritis is often six months. Occasionally, it is as long as 12 months. The researchers for this ACS study wanted to see how the patients did in the long term. They followed the research participants up to two years after their knee injections. The individuals who received hyaluronic acid injections continued to have the same pain as those who received a placebo. In constrast, those who received ACS remained improved—even after two years.[5] Later research also demonstrated that ACS was effective in treating OA pain in the hip[6] and rotator cuff tendons in the shoulder.[7] In these conditions, the results also appeared to be prolonged.

Why Does ACS Work Longer Term?

The long-lasting benefits of ACS couldn't be easily explained. I recall being at a conference several years ago when the speaker referred to ACS as "IRAP," standing for "IL-1Ra protein." The label presumed that ACS worked through IL-1Ra, quieting the effects of inflammatory IL-1. The problem with this theory was that a synthetic version of IL-1Ra had already been tested for individuals with knee OA. It didn't improve pain in the long term.[8] ACS was, therefore, unlikely to be working only through the actions of IL-1Ra.

Other scientists proposed that ACS, perhaps, worked through its collection of inflammation-resolving cytokines and growth factors. This was logical since IL-10, TGF, and other beneficial factors were also magnified. But these factors, like IL-1Ra, also had only short-term effects. None of these cytokine-blockers or growth factors could explain the prolonged pain relief that patients experienced. There was a piece of the puzzle still missing.

A few years ago, I began discussing these questions with Drs. Wehling and Reinecke in Germany and Dr. Ji at Duke's Center for Translational Pain Medicine. We decided to design a set of experiments to better understand the effects of ACS on (1) pain, (2) nerve inflammation, and (3) nerve function. As our experimental model, we chose to work with mice that had neuropathy from a chemotherapy drug called paclitaxel.

Paclitaxel, commonly used to treat breast and ovarian cancers, damages mitochondria and nerves. The more individuals are exposed to the chemotherapy, the worse the mitochondrial injury and the greater the nerve damage. With paclitaxel, nerve functions slow, nerve conduction velocities decrease, and the nerves become inflamed.

The effects of paclitaxel in mice can be accurately measured with several tools that Dr. Ji routinely used in his laboratory. To measure any impact from ACS, we also needed a control to use as a reference point and baseline. We decided to use serum that hadn't undergone extended clotting and incubation. We called the process of maintaining the serum under strict temperature and conditions an "incubation." The nonincubated serum contained normal proteins from the blood but lacked any factors unique to ACS.

Yul Huh, a PhD candidate in Dr. Ji's lab, performed the first experiments. He applied tiny filaments to the paws of the mice that had received the chemotherapy. The mice quickly pulled away, indicating they were experiencing skin sensitivity and nerve pain. Huh then injected either ACS or control serum into the mouse's spinal fluid and retested their paw sensitivity. The mice that received the nonincubated serum had no change. Their paws were as sensitive as before the injection. In constrast, the mice injected with ACS experienced immediate and significant pain relief.[9] Their paw sensitivity essentially went away.

The laboratory team followed and retested the mice twice a week to find out how long the effects of ACS lasted. They stopped testing after eight weeks, noting that the mice still had pain relief. The benefits of ACS lasted far beyond those seen with growth factors and inflammation-resolving cytokines. Something else was driving the effect.

We then ran experiments to determine the impact of ACS on nerve inflammation. Recall from Chapter 4, How Nerves (Mal)Function, that microglia in the spinal cord are like macrophages in the joints. They can become inflamed with injury. They can also "flip the switch" to an M2 cell and produce inflammation-resolving cytokines and anabolic growth factors. Fortunately, the inflammatory state of the microglia can be assessed with a microscope and special stains. We applied these stains to the spinal cords of mice that had received ACS and those that received control serum. The microglia of the mice who had received the control serum glowed with inflammation. Those that had received ACS had flipped their switch and become M2 cells. They were now resolving inflammation.

Nerve function in the mice was then tested by measuring nerve conduction velocities (described in Chapter 9, Exercise, Exosomes, and Reversing Neuropathy). After the mice received chemotherapy, their nerves slowed down, a sign of nerve damage and neuropathy. When mice were injected with ACS, their nerve velocities increased, indicating that their nerve function had improved. The ACS wasn't just reducing pain; it was reversing neuropathy.

Exosomes at Work

Although we saw prolonged reductions in pain and a speeding up of nerve velocities in the mice, we still didn't know what was providing these benefits. But we had a hunch. Immune cells under stress (such as exercise) release exosomes. Exosomes (Chapter 8, Exercise, Inflammation, and Joint Healing, and Chapter 9, Exercise, Exosomes, and Reversing Neuropathy) contain proteins, growth factors, and miRNAs that can control cell behavior. When miRNAs bind to messenger RNA (mRNA), they can stop the production of whatever protein the mRNA is going to make. Exosomes and their miRNAs have been shown to shut down destructive enzymes such as MMP in animal models of OA.[10] Exosomes have also been shown to improve nerve function and regrow small nerves in experimental neuropathy.[11] We needed to find out if exosomes played a role in ACS.

The first step was determining if ACS created exosomes. By collaborating with Dr. Tony Huang in Duke's Department of Engineering, we were able to use a specialized laser device to accomplish this. We found that ACS had approximately double the number of exosomes as the nonincubated serum. The extended clotting process released exosomes.

The next step was to determine if ACS-produced exosomes had a role in improving pain and nerve function in our chemotherapy-treated mice. The clearest way to understand the effects of the exosomes was to remove them and retest the exosome-free ACS in the mice. We reinjected the exosome-depleted ACS into the spinal fluid of mice with chemotherapy neuropathy. The mice got better, but only slightly. Taking out the exosomes decreased the effectiveness of the ACS by about 75 percent. The experiments were conclusive: The exosomes provided most of the benefits of ACS in treating our mice with chemotherapy neuropathy.

ACS for My Knee

After my second knee injury (introduced in Chapter 6, Igniting the Immune System to Heal), I exercised regularly. I did strength work to maintain the muscles, tendons, and ligaments and combined this routine with biking, jogging, and daily walks. Despite this program, I still experienced a nagging ache after a higher-intensity basketball game or tennis match. I had an X-ray done. Not surprisingly, it demonstrated some narrowing of the joint space of my knee in the same area where I had torn my meniscus. I had mild OA. With the meniscus injuries and prolonged release of inflammatory cytokines and catabolic enzymes, I had lost some cartilage. The pain I felt told me that this inflammatory and catabolic process was ongoing. I had a chronic wound that wouldn't heal.

At this point, I needed to decide whether to take a watch-and-wait approach or pursue a regenerative therapy. Inaction was less appealing after watching patients with similar injuries end up with knee replacements. I decided it was time to intervene. My goals were twofold. I wanted to play strenuous sports without stiffness and soreness afterward. More importantly, I wanted to protect my cartilage and avoid a future need for joint replacement surgery.

I knew the various options—PRP, MSCs, and ACS—in depth. I had researched all three of these interventions for years and routinely performed PRP and ACS injections in the clinic. With this knowledge, I was convinced that ACS would be my best option. After discussion and review of my MRI with Dr. Wehling, he agreed that I was a good candidate for ACS treatment. Since I had an upcoming medical conference in Amsterdam, I decided to take a couple extra days and visit his clinic in Düsseldorf, Germany.

I arrived at the clinic fresh off the plane and still bleary-eyed. Dr. Wehling gave me a tour of the clinic and laboratory. My prior visit was to learn how to offer ACS to my patients. During this visit, I was on the receiving end of the therapy. Dr. Wehling examined my knee, noting that the tendons and ligaments were strong. His assistant then drew my blood and sent it to the incubator, where my immune cells did their work. As my blood clotted, my platelets released their growth factors. Then, my macrophages morphed into M2 cells over subsequent hours and pumped out IL-1Ra, I-10, TGF, and other inflammation-resolving factors. Most importantly, this incubation process also released exosomes that would provide longer-term benefits for my knee cartilage.

Once the serum was processed, my knee was prepped with an antiseptic solution and injected. ACS is usually performed as a series of injections. Since I was traveling, I only had time for one injection. I was hoping that would be enough. I departed for the conference the next day. I walked around Amsterdam and biked into the countryside on beautiful Dutch bike paths that followed the rivers. I logged dozens of miles daily without swelling or pain (and sometimes left the conference early to enjoy the warm fall weather). At the week's close, I was ready to head home. The prolonged sitting on my flight from the US to Europe the previous week had resulted in quite a bit of knee soreness when I deplaned. I wasn't looking forward to the return trip. I boarded and settled in. Eight hours later, the plane landed at New York's JFK Airport, taxied to the gate, and the passengers slowly filed off. I stood up, anticipating the usual stiffness and pain. Except it wasn't there. My knee glided with complete smoothness. The difference from one flight to the next was remarkable.

The following week, I began to re-engage in higher-intensity sports. I started running longer distances and playing basketball with my fit 17-year-old son. These sports were enjoyable again. My stiffness and pain were gone. The immune imbalance was resolved. My wound had healed.

ACS, Exosomes, and Epigenetics

While anti-inflammatory cytokines and growth factors are essential components of regenerative therapies, exosomes are key to the prolonged effects of ACS. Exosomes promote tissue healing and help to resolve the chronic wounds of OA and neuropathy. Our research team saw this in the laboratory, and I felt it in my knee. ACS and exosomes affect epigenetics. They don't change the genetic code but they do change how cells read that code. The cells play the same piano (identical DNA), but the exosomes provide a different set of sheet music (miRNA changing the proteins made). The actions of exosomes explain the long-term benefits of ACS. As neurons and cartilage cells begin making new (and healthier) proteins, function is restored, and pain is reduced.

Takeaways

1. ACS is produced by turning on immune-based healing mechanisms of blood cells.
2. Clinical studies show the prolonged benefits of ACS in patients with osteoarthritis and sciatica.
3. Although ACS has inflammation-resolving cytokines and growth factors, experiments show that exosomes provide most benefits.

Chapter 15

Putting It All Together:
Immune Stimulation to Heal

The framework of how physicians understand a problem influences how we treat it. For instance, when osteoarthritis (OA) was framed as a "wear and tear" problem, recommendations followed to avoid impact exercise (that might worsen wear and tear). This framework and its recommendations were present until research showed that impact exercises can actually benefit our joints. The research prompted a framework shift and new recommendations to encourage impact exercise in *treating* OA.

In recent years, inflammation has emerged as the primary framework for understanding OA and neuropathy. Treatments again have followed the framework, with the development of multiple methods and medications to "fight" inflammation. Research is now teaching us another lesson. Studies have shown that suppressing inflammation can temporarily alleviate pain but does little to address the underlying cause of OA or neuropathy. Inflammation is present, but not the root cause of these diseases.

OA and neuropathy are best understood as chronic wounds that generate inflammation and pain. To improve these wounds, it is key to stimulate the immune cells to rebuild tissues and *resolve* the inflammation. Patients don't need to rush to the drugstore to buy the latest pharmaceuticals. The factors necessary for healing are already built into the immune systems. They simply need to be activated.

Making Regenerative Therapies Better

Regenerative therapies are potent tools to activate the body's own healing mechanisms, but inconsistencies still hinder them. There are dozens of devices used to make platelet-rich plasma (PRP), and the final products have little in common, except that they all come from blood. Some devices make platelet concentrations seven times (7X) greater than baseline. Others produce concentrations barely above the body's natural baseline. Unfortunately, all of these products are still called platelet-*rich* plasma, regardless of their contents. There have been several studies that show the importance of platelet concentrations for clinical effectiveness. It appears, unsurprisingly, that PRP must be rich in platelets to reduce the pain of knee OA.[1] While variety in the colors of fruits and vegetables is beneficial, variety in PRP is not. There needs to be greater consistency in PRP products to ensure effective results. Consistent results will also enable the medical community to advocate for insurance carriers to cover regenerative therapies to treat conditions such as OA. Given the current variability (and subsequent unsuccessful studies), insurance carriers can easily label PRP as "experimental" and deny coverage.

It is also important to establish consistency with MSCs, starting with their names. Referring to MSCs as "stem cells" causes confusion among patients (and physicians). As I described in Chapter 12, Are "Stem Cells" Really Stem Cells?, and Chapter 13, MSCs: Immune System Regulators, MSCs function through the immune system. They can be referred to as medicinal signaling cells, as Dr. Arnold Caplan suggested. Alternatively, they can be described based on their source: bone marrow concentrates, adipose concentrates, and so on. It is also important to indicate whether they have been cultured in a laboratory. There is a significant difference between bone marrow cells that are centrifuged and immediately injected and those cultured for weeks. Language is needed to clarify what kinds of cells doctors are preparing and injecting.

Another important distinction in regenerative therapies is whether they are sourced from the patients themselves (auto-biologic) or others (allobiologic). Therapies derived from the patients' own bodies should be prioritized whenever possible. Autobiologics reduce the risk of infection from donor tissues (such as amniotic, placental, or umbilical sources). They also minimize potential contamination that can occur during the processing of cells. Despite these risks, regenerative therapies from donor tissues will likely play a future role, particularly for individuals who do not respond to autobiologics. The challenge will be to identify those who will need these donor products. Doctors could use a "try and fail" approach. Inject PRP or other autobiologics first, and, if that doesn't work, move on to an allo-biologic. But this method is time-consuming, costly, and frustrating for patients. There needs to be a more effective way to predict an individual's response *before* the procedure.

As a physician, I can make some predictions. I know that PRP is less likely to relieve pain in someone with bone-on-bone OA. I can also predict that a regenerative therapy is less likely to help an individual who is not consuming healthy fats and plant color compounds. They don't have the raw materials that their immune cells need. But other outcomes are more challenging to forecast. A patient might be an excellent candidate with moderate OA, an exercise routine, and a diet of healthy foods. Yet, they still may not respond to a PRP injection. When this happens, the physician scratches their head in bewilderment, and the patient leaves frustrated. The opposite can also occur: A patient with bone-on-bone OA might experience months of improvement with a regenerative therapy, despite the doctor's lowered expectations. These surprises are likely due to a factor researchers have yet to measure.

Research on this "unmeasured factor" is being conducted in the laboratories of Dr. Luda Diatchenko at McGill University in Canada and Dr. Ru-Rong Ji in Duke's Anesthesiology Department. This factor likely involves the ability of immune cells to respond to stimuli. If immune cells, such as neutrophils and macrophages, cannot respond adequately to stimulation with regenerative therapies, individuals may experience limited pain relief from PRP and other autobiologics. Developing a clinical tool to assess "immune responsiveness" will require research funding and significant effort. Importantly, this research will not only provide a predictive tool for regenerative therapies but will also give insight into improving recovery from injury and reducing the risks of chronic pain. The medical community will learn which patients may regain immune function through exercise and healthy eating, and they will also discover which patients might benefit from extended clotting and immune stimulation treatments, such as ACS. Additionally, it will help to identify the subset of individuals who may require future allobiologic donor therapies. An immune-response tool will enable doctors to customize treatments for patients and determine the most effective ones *before* their application.

A Cell-Free Future?

The history of regenerative medicine is rich with cells. Cells from bone marrow. Cells from adipose tissue. Cells from umbilical cords that are grown in the laboratory. But as you learned in Chapters 12 and 13, these cells, such as MSCs, usually don't survive long-term after they're injected into a joint or around a nerve. These cells sacrifice themselves and alter the behavior of macrophages and other immune cells. As the immune response that promotes healing is increasingly better understood, the reliance on cells harvested from bone marrow, adipose, and other tissues will likely fade. An important cell-free trigger for a healing immune response has already been identified: exosomes. Exosomes are present throughout the body and are released by exercise and regenerative therapies such as autologous conditioned serum (ACS). Recall from Chapter 9, Exercise, Exosomes, and Reversing Neuropathy, that exosomes are only as effective as their cargo. Researchers continue to learn about their cargo's various components, including thousands of different proteins and miRNA. Several miRNAs have been identified that resolve inflammation and treat pain. Which methods of immune stimulation pack these exosomes with the most beneficial cargo are still to be determined.

The products derived from cells (rather than the cells themselves) will increasingly serve as tools for treating conditions such as OA and neuropathy. Cell-free autobiologic therapies, such as ACS, are already in use. Cell-free allobiologic therapies will also emerge. These donor treatments may come from cultured MSCs or other yet-to-be-identified sources. Safeguards will be necessary to ensure that donor products remain free from contamination. These cell-free therapies will continue to evolve as more is learned about the critical interactions between exosomes, growth factors, tissue repair, and the resolution of inflammation.

Healing Joints and Nerves

You might now ask, "What can I do now to engage these healing mechanisms for my own joints and nerves?" Below is a guide reflecting what I have learned from the laboratory, patients, and the thousand scientific papers I reviewed while writing this book. Also see Figure 15.1 on page 187 for a graphic showing the benefits of combining healthy foods, exercise, and regenerative therapies."

1. **Healthy Foods:**
   a. Focus on whole foods with no or minimal processing.
   b. Eat a wide variety of colorful vegetables and fruits. Those colors indicate the presence of flavonoids and other beneficial plant compounds.
   c. When possible, cook with extra-virgin olive or avocado oil.
   d. If you don't routinely eat cold-water fish (such as salmon, tuna, herring, anchovies, sardines, and others), consider taking an omega-3 supplement with at least 1,000 mg of combined DHA/EPA. Look for products certified to be free of contaminants such as heavy metals. Discuss starting any supplement with your medical professional.
   e. Choose nuts, such as walnuts, cashews, almonds, and dark chocolate for snacks.
   f. Enjoy teas, especially green teas that are rich in flavonoids.

2. **Exercise:**
   a. Combine endurance, strength, and balance exercises. Together, these activities stabilize joints, restore nerve function, and stimulate the immune system to improve tissue health.
   b. Exercise at least three to four times a week. Regular exercise produces growth factors, inflammation resolvers, and exosomes more efficiently.

c. Even if you are an experienced athlete, consider seeking the advice of a physical therapist or trainer. They can help you to build an injury-free exercise or recovery program.

d. Find your "Goldilocks" exercise routine and progress your workouts slowly. If you push so hard that you can't move the next day, you've pushed too hard. Give your body time to recover.

e. If joint or sciatica pain is holding you back from your exercise program, pursuing a single corticosteroid injection is okay. Sometimes an injection will get an individual "over the hump" and allow them to make longer-term progress. To minimize side effects, avoid repeated steroid injections.

f. Minimize NSAIDs and try to avoid taking them before exercise. Taking them before a workout blunts many of the tissue-building benefits of training.

3. **Regenerative therapies:**

a. If you are seeking information on regenerative therapies, speak with an experienced licensed physician or surgeon who can explain the pros and cons of these interventions *for you.*

b. Remember that regenerative therapies such as platelet-rich plasma (PRP) must stimulate the immune system to work. That means PRP must be rich in platelets (at least 3X baseline) to maximize benefits.

c. If you're considering medicinal signaling cells (MSCs; what many clinics call "stem cells"), ask your doctor if there are any advantages of MSCs over PRP *for you.* Many individuals with mild/moderate OA may do as well with PRP as MSCs.[2]

   d. If you are exploring allobiologic therapies, be cautious. Currently, there are no FDA-approved donor products. This means that outside of research protocols, the product you receive may not have been thoroughly tested for safety.

   e. If you are seeking autologous conditioned serum (ACS) as a treatment option, know it is only available in a limited number of US clinics that are licensed with the German parent company.

   f. Consider pursuing regenerative therapies before your OA or neuropathy is advanced. Prevention is easier than reversing disease.

Healthy foods, exercise, and regenerative therapies create a powerful healing combination. Together, these tools don't "fight" inflammation. They resolve it. Healthy fats and plant color compounds provide essential raw materials. Exercise stimulates the immune system. The regenerative therapies enhance and jump-start this entire process. Treatments containing exosomes take it a step further, reprogramming cells and improving the health of cartilage and neurons. The beauty of these interventions is that they don't suppress cell functions; they enrich them through the natural healing systems we've honed and perfected over millions of years. The tools to heal our joints and nerves are already within us.

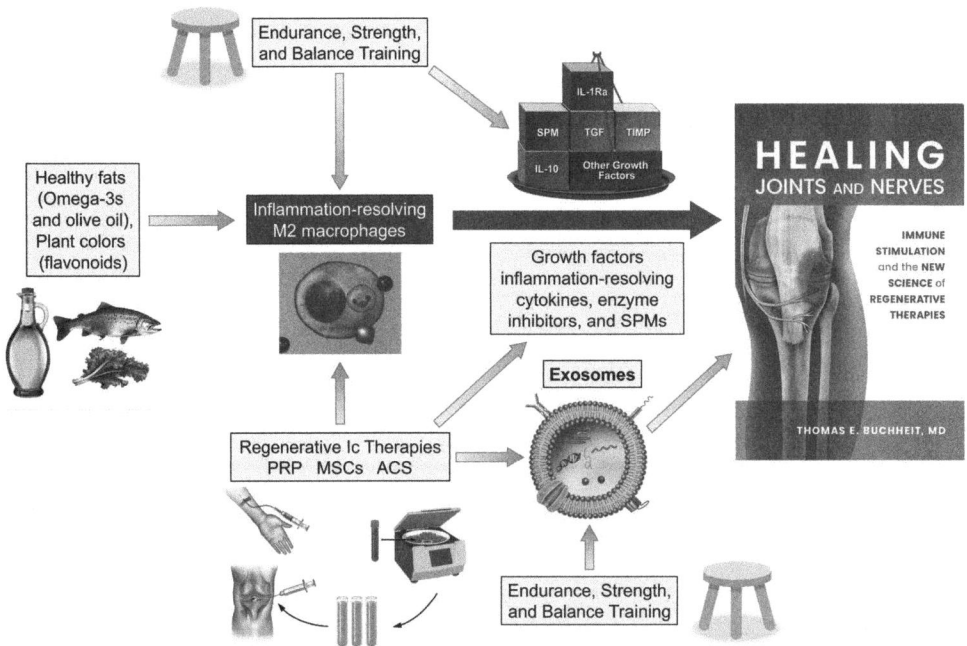

Figure 15.1. The benefits of combining healthy foods, exercise, and regenerative therapies: Foods provide the fuels and exercise "flips the switch" of the macrophage to begin resolving inflammation. When activated, M2 macrophage cells produce growth factors, inflammation-resolving cytokines, enzyme inhibitors, SPMs such as resolvins and protectins, and exosomes. If nutrition and exercise are not sufficient, regenerative therapies such as PRP, MSCs, and ACS can "jump start" these immune mechanisms. Together, these activities lead to the healing of joints and nerves.

Glossary

acetic acid: Acetic acid is a naturally occurring weak acid found in foods such as vinegar and sauerkraut.

ACS (autologous conditioned serum): This autobiologic therapy is produced by blood and immune cells that undergo extended clotting and immune stimulation. ACS contains growth factors, inflammation-resolving cytokines, and exosomes.

adipose tissue: Adipose tissue contains multiple cell types, including adipose (fat) cells that serve as energy storage, and a smaller percentage of MSCs (medicinal signaling cells). MSCs from adipose tissue are sometimes isolated or cultured to alleviate osteoarthritis pain.

allobiologic/allogenic product: Allobiologic products refer to blood, cells, or tissues donated from one individual and given to another. In scientific publications, allobiologics are commonly referred to as "allogenic biologics."

amino acid: Amino acids are the building blocks for proteins. There are 20 amino acids that the human body use to produce more than 100,000 different kinds of proteins.

anabolic: Anabolic substances promote the building and repair of tissues. Anabolic proteins in the body include multiple types of growth factors, which are released by exercise and regenerative therapies.

analgesic: Analgesics are medications or natural compounds that relieve pain. Willow bark, aspirin, and NSAIDs are all anti-inflammatories (reducing inflammation) and analgesics (relieving pain).

antibodies: Antibodies are proteins produced by immune cells that bind tightly to markers on the surface of viruses, bacteria, and sometimes the body's own cells. Precise targeting of antibodies is used to manufacture drugs that treat rheumatoid arthritis by suppressing TNF and IL-1.

anticoagulation: Anticoagulation involves using a medication or chemical to prevent blood from forming a clot. Anticoagulants are added to platelet-rich plasma and MSCs during processing and allow the cells to separate by weight in a centrifuge.

ATP (adenosine triphosphate): ATP is the molecule that provides energy for active processes in all the cells of the body. Most of the ATP in the body is produced in the mitochondria.

autobiologic: Autobiologics are blood, cells, or tissues that come from and return to the same individual. An autobiologic contrasts with an allo-biologic (where donor and recipient are different individuals). In scientific publications, autobiologics are commonly referred to as "autologous biologics."

autoimmune conditions: In autoimmune conditions, such as rheumatoid arthritis, the body reacts against itself. Autoimmune conditions can produce significant concentrations of inflammatory cytokines such as TNF and IL-1.

autophagy: Autophagy is the process a cell uses to recycle its parts. During autophagy, cell organelles fuse with a lysosome, and their parts are broken down and recycled.

axon: An axon is the part of a neuron that conducts electrical impulses away from the cell body. Axons in the sciatic nerve extend from the lower back down to the foot.

bone marrow: Bone marrow contains cells that generate the red blood cells, leukocytes, and platelets that circulate in blood. Bone marrow, especially in the pelvis, also contains a small percentage of MSCs. MSCs from bone marrow have been grown in the laboratory and are used to treat conditions such as osteoarthritis pain.

carbohydrates: Carbohydrates are carbon molecules, such as glucose, that serve as an energy source for cells and their mitochondria. Carbohydrate chains, such as keratin and chondroitin, are also components of proteoglycans and provide cushion in cartilage.

cartilage: Cartilage is the smooth, resilient surface of bones that allows people to move their joints without resistance. Cartilage is made of tough collagen fibers mixed with large cushioning proteoglycan molecules. Cartilage has no nerve supply or sensation.

catabolic: A catabolic process breaks down tissues. Chronic exposure of cartilage to inflammatory cytokines such as IL-1 and TNF is catabolic, leading to the development of osteoarthritis.

cell body: The cell body is the central part of a neuron that contains the DNA and protein manufacturing machinery. The cell bodies for sciatic neurons are located near the lower spine. Cell bodies manufacture proteins that are transported down the long axons of the sciatic nerve.

cell membrane: The membrane is the coating around a cell that separates the cell contents from its surroundings. A cell membrane is made of proteins and fats. The stiffness of the cell membrane is affected by the kinds of fats that a person consumes.

cell nucleus: The cell nucleus contains DNA and protein manufacturing machinery. The nucleus of a neuron is located in the cell body.

central nervous system: The central nervous system contains the brain and spinal cord.

centrifuge: A centrifuge is a device that spins test tubes at high speeds and generates significant gravitational forces. A centrifuge is used to separate different cell types in platelet-rich plasma and MSC therapies.

chemotherapy: Chemotherapy drugs are chemical compounds used to treat cancers. Some, such as paclitaxel, also damage mitochondria. The mitochondrial injury from paclitaxel reduces nerve function and can cause pain and weakness, especially in the feet.

collagen: Collagen is made up of long protein strands that provide structure and strength to multiple tissues, such as cartilage, tendons, bone, and skin. Collagen is mixed with proteoglycan to form the cartilage of joints.

corticosteroid: Corticosteroids are inflammation-suppressing compounds that the body produces in the adrenal glands. Synthetic corticosteroids are commonly injected to treat the pain associated with osteoarthritis and neuropathy.

cortisol: Cortisol is a naturally occurring corticosteroid from the adrenal glands. Cortisol was one of the original corticosteroids isolated from cows and injected into patients to treat the inflammation and pain of rheumatoid arthritis.

COX-1 enzymes: COX stands for cyclooxygenase. COX enzymes produce lipids called prostaglandins. There are two types of COX enzymes in the body: COX-1 and COX-2. COX-1 enzymes make prostaglandins that perform vital functions, such as protecting the stomach and maintaining blood flow to the kidneys. Many NSAIDs partially block COX-1 enzymes and can lead to stomach and kidney side effects if taken for extended periods.

COX-2 enzymes: COX-2 enzymes produce prostaglandins involved in inflammation and pain. These enzymes are blocked by a group of NSAIDs called COX-2 inhibitors, such as celecoxib and meloxicam.

Crohn's disease: Crohn's disease is an autoimmune disease associated with high levels of inflammatory cytokines such as TNF and IL-1. Crohn's affects the digestive tract and is commonly treated with potent cytokine suppressors.

cytokine: Cytokines are small proteins released from immune cells that regulate all aspects of immune function and inflammation. Some cytokines, such as IL-1 and TNF, are catabolic and break down tissues if released for prolonged periods of time. Others, such as IL-1Ra and IL-10, are critical for the resolution of inflammation and healing.

diabetes: Diabetes disease causes chronic elevations of glucose that can damage mitochondria and reduce the energy supply to neurons. Diabetes is the most common cause of neuropathy in the US.

disc herniation: A disc herniation occurs when a spine disc experiences a tear in its cartilage ring and the gelatinous nucleus in the center of the disc extrudes and puts pressure on the spinal nerves. Disc herniations can cause significant inflammation and pain of the spinal nerves, leading to sciatica.

DNA (deoxyribonucleic acid): DNA makes up the genetic code of human cells. DNA is copied to messenger RNA (mRNA), which is used to synthesize proteins. By splicing and recombining mRNAs, the same DNA segment can produce several different types of proteins. Epigenetics regulates how DNA is utilized and the kinds of proteins that are produced.

DNA methylation: When methyl groups (carbon atoms bound to hydrogen) are added to specific sections of DNA, the mRNA copying machinery is prevented from attaching, silencing genes and preventing them from creating proteins. Each cell type in the body has a different DNA methylation pattern that defines its function. The DNA methylation pattern of cells changes with age and can be analyzed in the laboratory. Analysis of DNA methylation patterns is one of the methods used to determine an individual's epigenetic age.

elastin: Elastins are long, flexible proteins in tendons, blood vessels, and skin that provide stretch. In tendons, this stretch buffers the forces between muscle and bone and offers protection from injury during jumps and falls.

enzymes: Enzymes are specialized proteins that speed up chemical reactions in the body. Enzymes help to digest food, make energy in the mitochondria, and carry out cell functions necessary for life. Some enzymes, such as MMP, can break down tissues and damage cartilage in joints with osteoarthritis.

epidural steroid injection: The injection of corticosteroid into the spinal canal and around the spinal nerves. Epidural steroid injections are used to treat the nerve inflammation and pain associated with disc herniations and spinal stenosis.

epigenetics: Epigenetics controls which genes are turned on and off to make a protein. Epigenetic mechanisms, such as histone protein modification, DNA methylation, and microRNAs (miRNAs), determine how a cell develops and its health over time. Multiple factors, including diet and exercise, affect which epigenetic mechanisms are activated.

exosomes: Exosomes are tiny communication vesicles found in blood, spinal fluid, breast milk, and all tissues of the body. Exosomes change the behavior and function of recipient cells, including neurons, cartilage cells, and immune cells. The effects of exosomes vary widely and depend on their sources and contents.

fats: Fats are collections of different kinds of fatty acids. Fats that contain a large percentage of saturated fatty acids are often solid at room temperature. Fats that contain monounsaturated and polyunsaturated fatty acids are often liquid at room temperature and are commonly called oils.

fatty acids: Fatty acids serve as fuel for mitochondria when their long carbon chains are broken down into smaller fragments. Fatty acids are also used by the body to manufacture lipids that control inflammation and its resolution. The three main types of fatty acids are saturated, monounsaturated, and polyunsaturated.

FGF (fibroblast growth factor): A growth factor released by platelets that stimulates cartilage cell growth. FGF has been tested as a treatment for osteoarthritis. This growth factor appears to protect cartilage from damage but does not significantly improve pain.

flavonoid: Flavonoid compounds give fruits, vegetables, and berries their deep red, blue, purple, orange, and green hues. Flavonoids provide many of the health benefits of these plants. Flavonoids act as scavengers, clearing out the damaging high-energy particles that escape from injured mitochondria. Flavonoids also enhance the production of inflammation-resolving SPMs, such as resolvins and protectins.

fluorescent cell: When cells are treated with fluorescent dyes, they emit light which is visible to specialized microscopes. Fluorescent cells are used in stem cell research to determine where cells migrate and how long they live after injection.

gene expression: Gene expression—the process of making proteins from DNA genes—has two primary steps. First, DNA is copied and spliced to messengerRNA. Next, the mRNA serves as a blueprint to assemble amino acids into proteins. Gene expression is controlled by epigenetics.

glial cell: Glial cells surround neurons in the brain and peripheral nervous system. Glial cells such as microglia carry out immune functions. Other glial cells, such as Schwann cells, provide protective functions and speed nerve transmission.

growth factor (GF): Growth factors are proteins released from platelets and immune cells that help build and repair tissues. Most growth factors are anabolic, promoting tissue strength and health.

histone proteins: Histone proteins serve as structural support for DNA in the nucleus of a cell. Histone proteins can be modified by adding or subtracting molecules. If molecules are removed, DNA wraps more tightly, and the mRNA copying machinery cannot access the DNA gene. If molecules are added to histone proteins, DNA loosens, allowing it to be copied to mRNA and made into proteins. There are multiple regulators of histone proteins, including sirtuins.

hyaluronic acid (HA): A large molecule that provides lubrication for joint fluid and cushion for joint cartilage. With osteoarthritis, hyaluronic acid molecules break down into smaller fragments, causing joint stiffness and chronic inflammation.

IL-1: IL-1 is an inflammatory cytokine that can cause joint and nerve pain. Chronic exposure to IL-1 causes cartilage to break down and osteoarthritis to develop.

IL-1Ra: IL-1Ra stands for "IL-1 receptor antagonist." It opposes the effects of IL-1, resolving inflammation and reducing pain. IL-1Ra is released by M2 macrophages and is found in high concentrations in ACS.

IL-6: IL-6 is an inflammatory cytokine similar to IL-1 and TNF. Chronically high levels of IL-6 can cause pain and cartilage breakdown. IL-6 is also released in short bursts with exercise. IL-6 can act as an immune stimulant, helping macrophages "flip the switch" to an M2 cell and begin resolving inflammation.

IL-10: IL-10 is a cytokine with inflammation-resolving effects. IL-10 is released by M2 macrophages and can reduce pain.

interferon: Interferon proteins are released by immune cells in response to infection. Interferons cause aches and stimulate the immune system. Laboratory research has demonstrated that some types of interferons can resolve chronic pain.

interleukins: Interleukin proteins act as messengers between leukocytes and other immune cells. Some interleukins can produce inflammation (such as IL-1 and IL-6), and others are inflammation resolving (such as IL-1Ra and IL-10).

leukocyte: Also called white blood cells, leukocytes include neutrophils, monocytes, macrophages, M2 macrophages, and other immune-active cells in the blood. Leukocytes play a crucial role in the healing cascade and the resolution of inflammation.

leukocyte-rich PRP: PRP is considered to be leukocyte-rich when the concentration of leukocytes in the PRP product is greater than the baseline leukocyte concentration of a patient's blood. Leukocytes in PRP can cause an acute inflammatory reaction after injection. Leukocyte-rich PRP can also stimulate the body's healing cascade.

lipids: Lipids are a broad class of organic compounds that do not dissolve in water. There are multiple types of lipids, such as fatty acids, prostaglandins, and corticosteroids. Some lipids are consumed as food. Others, including resolvins and protectins, are manufactured by cells in the body.

lysosome: Lysosomes are organelles in the cell that contain enzymes, which can digest cell parts. Lysosomes are essential tools that clean up and recycle malfunctioning cell parts in a process called autophagy.

M2 macrophage (M2 Cell): After a macrophage is activated, it can transition from an inflammatory cell to an M2 cell. The M2 macrophage cell releases multiple inflammation-resolving cytokines, such as IL-1Ra and IL-10, which can also reduce pain. Exercise and the regenerative therapies stimulate the transition of the inflammatory macrophage to the inflammation-resolving M2 macrophage.

macrophages: Macrophage immune cells are critically important for resolving inflammation. When activated, macrophages initially secrete inflammatory proteins and cytokines, such as IL-1 and TNF. After 1–2 days of inflammation, a macrophage can "flip its switch" to an M2 macrophage and begin the process of resolving inflammation and rebuilding tissues.

MSC: MSC originally stood for "mesenchymal stem cell" and described a type of bone marrow cell that could be cultured and grown in the laboratory to form cartilage, bone, or adipose tissue. Research has demonstrated that MSCs don't work by growing new cartilage, but by stimulating the M2 macrophage to resolve inflammation and improve pain. Reflecting this new understanding, MSC now commonly stands for "medicinal signaling cell."

meta-analysis: Meta-analysis combines the results of multiple studies on the same topic or intervention. A meta-analysis can sometimes detect effects that might not be seen in smaller studies.

metabolic disease: Metabolic diseases are disorders that disrupt the body's normal energy-producing chemical reactions. One of the most common metabolic diseases is diabetes, in which mitochondria are damaged, preventing efficient use of fuel sources like glucose.

microglia: A microglia is a glial cell that surrounds neurons, especially in the spinal cord and brain. Microglia originate from the same cell line as macrophages (in the joints) and function in a similar manner. When activated, microglia release IL-1, TNF, and other inflammatory cytokines. Microglia can also "flip the switch" to an M2 cell and begin the process of resolving inflammation and reducing pain.

miRNA (microRNA): miRNAs are an important epigenetic mechanism that controls which mRNAs survive to be copied into proteins. When an miRNA binds to its matching mRNA, it neutralizes or destroys the mRNA. miRNAs control immune function, response to injury, and recovery. Several hundred different kinds of miRNAs are contained in exosomes.

mitochondrion: The organelle in the cell that creates energy in the form of ATP. Mitochondria take glucose and fatty acid fragments and use them to generate high-energy electrons and protons. The high-energy protons are shunted to the outer part of the mitochondria, creating a batterylike gradient that generates large quantities of ATP. When mitochondria are injured, they can leak their high-energy particles, damaging neurons and other cells.

MMP enzymes: MMP stands for matrix metalloproteinase. MMP concentrations increase in joints and nerves after prolonged exposure to inflammatory cytokines such as IL-1 and TNF. Excesses of MMP damage the collagen and proteoglycans in cartilage.

monocyte: A monocyte is an immune cell in the blood that becomes a macrophage with tissue damage. After injury, monocytes squeeze through broken blood vessels and morph into giant macrophages that release multiple inflammatory proteins and jump-start the healing cascade.

MRI (magnetic resonance imaging): An MRI is an imaging tool used to assess soft tissues such as joint cartilage, tendons, ligaments, and lumbar discs. Modern MRIs generate tremendously detailed images, including minor abnormalities that may not always be of functional importance. MRIs should be reviewed in the context of a patient's function and symptoms.

mRNA (messenger ribonucleic acid): mRNA is copied and spliced from DNA gene segments and serves as a blueprint for the manufacturing of proteins. Multiple mRNAs can be made from the same DNA gene, producing a diversity of proteins.

myelin: Myelin is the protective coating on neurons produced by Schwann cells. Myelin, and its gaps called nodes of Ranvier, significantly speed up nerve conduction velocity.

myositis: Myositis refers to any inflammation of muscle tissue. Myositis can accompany autoimmune diseases that release high concentrations of IL-1, TNF, and other inflammatory cytokines.

nerve conduction velocity: Nerve conduction velocities measure nerve speed. Velocity is tested by electrically stimulating a nerve at one location and measuring the time it takes for the nerve signal to reach a second location. Individuals with exposure to chemotherapy, diabetes, or other causes of neuropathy often experience a decrease in nerve conduction velocity.

nerve fiber density: This test for neuropathy takes a skin biopsy and treats it with a stain that only affects nerves. When the skin is viewed under a microscope, small nerves can be counted, and nerve density is calculated. Nerve fiber density decreases in many neuropathies as the ends of nerves die.

neuron: Neurons are the individual cells that make up nerves. Neurons have a cell body that contains the nucleus and DNA, and an axon that projects outward from the cell body.

neuropathy: Neuropathy refers to an injury to the nervous system. This term is often used interchangeably with peripheral neuropathy, which describes damage to the peripheral nerves. Neuropathy frequently occurs with diseases such as diabetes and after exposure to toxins like chemotherapy. It causes symptoms of numbness and pain, particularly in the feet. Neuropathy is sometimes assessed by testing nerve conduction velocities and nerve fiber densities.

neutrophil: Neutrophils are white blood cells that are often the first to arrive at an area of tissue injury. Neutrophils clean up debris and remove bacterial invaders. These immune cells also release multiple inflammatory cytokines and recruit monocytes/macrophages to the area to start the healing cascade.

nodes of Ranvier: The nodes of Ranvier are gaps in the myelin coating of neurons. When a neuron fires, sodium channels open, creating an electrical current that rolls down the neuron. If a neuron has myelin and nodes of Ranvier, the electrical current can jump from node to node, speeding up the electrical current.

NSAID: NSAID stands for nonsteroidal anti-inflammatory drug and describes multiple medications that patients take to reduce pain. NSAIDs turn off COX enzymes and reduce the production of inflammatory prostaglandins.

omega-3: Omega-3 fatty acids are a type of polyunsaturated fatty acid found in fish, nuts, and some seeds, such as flaxseed. Omega-3 fatty acids are metabolized by the body to SPMs, such as resolvins and protectins, that resolve inflammation and reduce pain.

omega-6: Omega-6 fatty acids are a type of polyunsaturated fatty acid found in many seeds and vegetables. The body does not manufacture omega-6 fatty acids, and people must get omega-6s from their diet. In addition to using omega-6s as a fuel source for mitochondria, the body can also convert these fatty acids into inflammatory prostaglandins. Laboratory research has demonstrated that excessive intake of omega-6 fatty acids can lead to joint inflammation and decreases in nerve health.

organelle: An organelle is a specialized structure within the cell that carries out a specific function. Examples of organelles include mitochondria and lysosomes. Mitochondria generate energy in the form of ATP. Lysosomes digest unhealthy mitochondria to recycle their parts and improve cell health.

osteoarthritis (OA): OA is a painful joint condition diagnosed by narrowing of the space between bones as shown on X-ray. Caused by chronic elevation of inflammatory cytokines and the release of enzymes such as MMP that break down the components of cartilage, OA decreases the health and thickness of cartilage and causes bone spurs.

paclitaxel: Paclitaxel is a chemotherapy used to treat breast, lung, and colon cancer. Paclitaxel injures mitochondria, slows the transport of proteins and nutrition in neurons, and can cause painful neuropathy.

peripheral nervous system: The peripheral nervous system is the part of the nervous system outside of the brain and spinal cord. Large peripheral nerves include the sciatic nerve (in the leg) and the median nerve (in the arm/wrist).

platelet-derived growth factor (PDGF): PDGF is a growth factor found in platelets and released at times of injury that stimulates cell growth, including the growth of cartilage cells. PDGF is concentrated in platelet-rich plasma and other regenerative therapies.

platelet-rich plasma (PRP): PRP is created by spinning blood in a centrifuge and allowing the platelets and cells to separate by gravity. PRP is the part of plasma that contains high concentrations of platelets and variable concentrations of leukocytes. PRP is commonly used to stimulate an immune response and treat osteoarthritis.

platelets: Platelets are small cell fragments in the blood that cause clots to form. Platelets also contain hundreds of growth factors that are released at the time of injury and stimulate tissue growth and recovery.

prostaglandin: Prostaglandins are lipids that control multiple essential functions in the body, including the regulation of blood flow and the control of inflammation. Excesses of inflammatory prostaglandins can lead to worsened joint pain and nerve malfunction. The body's production of inflammatory prostaglandins is reduced by NSAIDs.

protectins: Protectins are specialized pro-resolving mediators (SPMs) derived from omega-3 fatty acids. Protectins are manufactured and released by immune cells such as the M2 macrophage. These SPMs protect nerves at times of injury or stress and reduce pain.

protein: Proteins are large molecules built from amino acids according to a blueprint determined by mRNA. Proteins are involved in nearly all structures and functions in the body. They make up vital components of joint cartilage, tendons, and ligaments. Proteins, such as cytokines, also control immune system function and regulate inflammation. The body has over 100,000 different kinds of proteins.

proteoglycan: Proteoglycans are giant cushioning molecules that combine with collagen to make hyaline cartilage for joints. Proteoglycan contains hyaluronic acid and large carbohydrate molecules, such as keratin and chondroitin. With osteoarthritis, enzymes can break down the components of proteoglycan, leading to the thinning and loss of cartilage health.

red blood cells: Red blood cells in the blood carry oxygen to tissues. Red blood cells are heavier than other types of blood cells, allowing them to be easily separated by the gravitational forces of a centrifuge.
In a centrifuge, red blood cells settle to the bottom of the test tube.

regenerative therapy: Regenerative therapies restore damaged or diseased tissues. Most successful regenerative therapies stimulate the body's immune cells. These treatments, such as platelet-rich plasma, MSCs, and autologous conditioned serum, help the body self-repair.

resolvins: Resolvins are specialized pro-resolving mediators (SPMs) derived from omega-3 fatty acids. Resolvins and protectins are manufactured and released by immune cells such as the M2 macrophage. These SPMs resolve inflammation and reduce pain without disrupting the healing cascade.

rheumatoid arthritis (RA): RA is an autoimmune condition that produces high concentrations of inflammatory cytokines, such as IL-1 and TNF, in the joints. If left unchecked, these cytokines will cause joint swelling and break down cartilage. RA usually improves with drugs that suppress IL-1 and TNF.

Schwann cells: Schwann cells are a type of glial cell that surrounds most of the peripheral nerves in the body. Schwann cells support the health of neurons through vesicles such as exosomes. Schwann cells also speed up nerve conduction velocity, allowing rapid coordination of activities.

sciatica: Sciatica is pain caused by damage or inflammation of the sciatic nerve or the spinal nerves that make up the sciatic. A common cause of sciatica is compression of nerves from a disc herniation or spinal stenosis. Symptoms include shooting and burning pain, and sometimes numbness. The ends of the sciatic nerve in the feet are particularly susceptible to damage because of the physical distance from their cell bodies, which are located in the lower spine.

sensory nerve: Sensory nerves carry sensations such as touch and temperature from hands, feet, and other body areas to the spinal cord and brain. Sensory nerves are not simple tubes carrying messages, but complex, branching structures with connections that can strengthen with repeated use.

sirtuins: Sirtuins are a group of important histone protein regulators. Sirtuin proteins are epigenetic controllers that determine which segments of DNA are unwrapped from their histone proteins and are available for copying to mRNA.

spinal stenosis: Stenosis involves narrowing of the canal and the holes where spinal nerves exit. Stenosis is a slow process commonly caused by arthritis in the spine and the development of bone spurs. If stenosis becomes severe, it can cause inflammation and pain in spinal nerves.

SPM: SPM stands for specialized pro-resolving mediators. SPMs are a group of lipids—including resolvins and protectins—that immune cells, such as M2 macrophages, produce from omega-3 fatty acids in the diet. SPMs resolve inflammation.

stem cells: This term refers to cells that can grow and develop into different types of tissues. There are several different types of stem cells including: (1) embryonic stem cells that can create an entire human or animal;

(2) blood stem cells which generate leukocytes, platelets, and red blood cells; and (3) mesenchymal "stem cells" or MSCs, which can produce bone, muscle, cartilage, and adipose in the laboratory. Many scientists argue that MSCs should be described as "medicinal signaling cells" rather than stem cells.

TGF (transforming growth factor): TGF is a growth factor produced by platelets and M2 macrophages that promotes tissue recovery. TGF produces pain relief with the injection of regenerative therapies, such as platelet-rich plasma, MSCs, and ACS.

TNF (tumor necrosis factor): TNF is an inflammatory cytokine with similar effects as IL-1, causing worsened joint and nerve pain. Chronic exposure to TNF causes cartilage to break down and osteoarthritis to develop.

ultrasound: A medical diagnostic tool that uses high frequency sound waves to visualize anatomic structures under the skin, ultrasound is an effective tool to assess the health of tissues such as ligaments, tendons, and nerves. It is most effective in visualizing structures near the skin surface such as the rotator cuff of the shoulder and the peripheral nerves near the hands and feet.

vesicle: Vesicles are membrane-bound sacs that contain cell contents. Vesicles can be inside the cell, such as the lysosome, or outside the cell, such as the exosome. The membrane of a vesicle protects its contents from being degraded.

white blood cells: Also called leukocytes, white blood cells include neutrophils, monocytes, macrophages, and other immune-active cells in the blood. White blood cells play a crucial role in the healing cascade and the resolution of inflammation.

Notes

Chapter 1

1 H. Song, J. Zhao, J. Cheng, et al. "Extracellular Vesicles in Chondrogenesis and Cartilage Regeneration." *Journal of Cellular and Molecular Medicine* 25 (2021): 4883–92, https://doi.org/10.1111/jcmm.16290.

2 S. G. F. Abram, A. Judge, D. J. Beard, A. J. Carr, AND A. J. Price. "Long-Term Rates of Knee Arthroplasty in a Cohort of 834 393 Patients with a History of Arthroscopic Partial Meniscectomy." *Bone & Joint Journal* 101-b, no. 9 (2019): 1071–80, https://doi.org/10.1302/0301-620x.101b9.Bjj-2019-0335.R1; F. W. Roemer, C. K. Kwoh, M. J. Hannon, et al. "Partial Meniscectomy Is Associated with Increased Risk of Incident Radiographic Osteoarthritis and Worsening Cartilage Damage in the Following Year." *European Radiology* 27 (2017): 404–13, https://doi.org/10.1007/s00330-016-4361-z.

3 S. F. Kane, L. H. Olewinski, and K. S. Tamminga. "Management of Chronic Tendon Injuries." *American Family Physician* 100, no. 3 (2019): 147–57, https://pubmed.ncbi.nlm.nih.gov/31361101.

4 D. Docheva, S. A. Muller, M. Majewski, and C. H. Evans. "Biologics for Tendon Repair." *Advanced Drug Delivery Reviews* 84 (2015) (2015): 222–239. https://doi.org/10.1016/j.addr.2014.11.015.

5 S. P. Magnusson and M. Kjaer. "The Impact of Loading, Unloading, Ageing and Injury on the Human Tendon." *Journal of Physiology* 597, no. 5 (2019): 1283–98, https://doi.org/10.1113/jp275450.

6 K. Yamakado. "The Targeting Accuracy of Subacromial Injection to the Shoulder: An Arthrographic Evaluation." *Arthroscopy* 18, no. 8 (2002): 887–91, https://doi.org/10.1053/jars.2002.35263.

Chapter 2

1 E. A. Carswell, L. J. Old, R. L. Kassel, and B. Williamson. "An Endotoxin-Induced Serum Factor That Causes Necrosis of

Tumors." *Proceedings of the National Academy of Sciences* 72, no. 9
(1975): 3666–70, https://doi.org/10.1073/pnas.72.9.3666.

2   N. J. Roberts, S. Zhou, L. A. Diaz Jr., and M. Holdhoff. "Systemic
Use of Tumor Necrosis Factor Alpha as an Anticancer Agent."
Oncotarget 2 (2011): 739–51, https://doi.org/10.18632/oncotarget
.344.

3   M. J. Elliott, N. M. Ravinder, M. Feldmann, et al. "Treatment of
Rheumatoid Arthritis with Chimeric Monoclonal Antibodies
to Tumor Necrosis Factor Alpha." *Arthritis & Rheumatology* 36
(1993): 1681–90, https://doi.org/10.1002/art.1780361206.

4   S. Perez-Garcia, M. Carrión, Irene Gutiérrez-Cañas, et al. "Profile
of Matrix-Remodeling Proteinases in Osteoarthritis: Impact of
Fibronectin." *Cells* 9, no. 1 (2020): 40, https://doi.org/10.3390
/cells9010040; G. A. Homandberg, Y. Kang, J. Zhang, A. A. Cole, ,
and J. M. Williams. "A Single Injection of Fibronectin Fragments
into Rabbit Knee Joints Enhances Catabolism in the Articular
Cartilage Followed by Reparative Responses but also Induces
Systemic Effects in the Non-Injected Knee Joints." *Osteoarthritis
Cartilage* 9 (2001): 673–83, https://doi.org/10.1053/joca.2001.0419.

5   X. Chevalier, P. Goupille, A. D. Beaulieu, et al. "Intraarticular
Injection of Anakinra in Osteoarthritis of the Knee: A Multicenter,
Randomized, Double-Blind, Placebo-Controlled Study." *Arthritis &
Rheumatism* 61, no. 3 (2009): 344–52, https://doi.org/10.1002
/art.24096.

6   M. Kloppenburg, R. Ramonda, K. Bobacz, et al. "Etanercept in
Patients with Inflammatory Hand Osteoarthritis (EHOA):
A Multicentre, Randomised, Double-Blind, Placebo-Controlled
Trial." *Annals of the Rheumatic Diseases* 77, no. 12: (2018): 1757–64,
https://doi.org/10.1136/annrheumdis-2018-213202; D. Aitken,
L. L. Laslett, F. Pan, et al. "A Randomised Double-Blind Placebo-
Controlled Crossover Trial of HUMira (Adalimumab) for Erosive
Hand OsteoaRthritis—The HUMOR Trial." *Osteoarthritis and
Cartilage* 26, no. 7 (2018): 880–87, https://doi.org/10.10161
/j.joca.2018.02.899.

7   M. T. Hannan, D. T. Felson, and T. Pincus. "Analysis of the
Discordance Between Radiographic Changes and Knee Pain in
Osteoarthritis of the Knee." *Journal of Rheumatology* 27, no. 6
(2000): 1513–17. https://pubmed.ncbi.nlm.nih.gov/10852280.

8 F. Birrell, M. Lunt, G. Macfarlane, and A. Silman. "Association Between Pain in the Hip Region and Radiographic Changes of Osteoarthritis: Results from a Population-Based Study." *Rheumatology (Oxford)* 44, no. 3 (2005): 337–41, https://doi .org/10.1093/rheumatology/keh458.

9 J. S. Sher, J. W. Uribe, A. Posada, B. J. Murphy, and M. B. Zlatkin. "Abnormal Findings on Magnetic Resonance Images of Asymptomatic Shoulders." *Journal of Bone & Joint Surgery* 77, no. 1 (1995): 10–15, https://doi.org/10.2106/00004623-199501000 -00002.

10 E. Sanchez-Lopez, R. Coras, A. Torres, N. E. Lane, and M. Guma. "Synovial Inflammation in Osteoarthritis Progression." *Nature Reviews Rheumatology* 18 (2022): 258–75, https://doi.org/10.1038 /s41584-022-00749-9.

Chapter 3

1 J.-P. Auger, M. Zimmermann, M. Faas, et al. "Metabolic Rewiring Promotes Anti-Inflammatory Effects of Glucocorticoids." *Nature* (2024): 184–92, https://doi.org/10.1038/s41586-024-07282-7.

2 T. G. Benedek. "History of the Development of Corticosteroid Therapy." *Clinical and Exxperimental Rheumatology* 29, supp. 68 (2011): S5–12, https://pubmed.ncbi.nlm.nih.gov/22018177.

3 J. L. Hollander, E. M. Brown Jr., R. A. Jessar, and C. Y. Brown. "Hydrocortisone and Cortisone Injected into Arthritic Joints; Comparative Effects of and Use of Hydrocortisone as a Local Antiarthritic Agent." *JAMA* 147, no. 17 (1951): 1629–35, https://doi.org/10.1001/jama.1951.03670340019005.

4 A. Al-Shoha, D. S. Rao, J. Schilling, E. Peterson, and S. Mandel. "Effect of Epidural Steroid Injection on Bone Mineral Density and Markers of Bone Turnover in Postmenopausal Women." *Spine* 37, no. 25 (2012): E1567–71, https://doi.org/10.1097/BRS .0b013e318270280e.

5 A. S. Wang, E. J. Armstrong, and A. W. Armstrong. "Corticosteroids and Wound Healing: Clinical Considerations in the Perioperative Period." *American Journal of Surgery* 206, no. 3 (2013): 410–17, https://doi.org/10.1016/j.amjsurg.2012.11.018.

6 T. E. McAlindon, M. P. LaValley, W. F. Harvey, et al. "Effect of Intra-Articular Triamcinolone vs Saline on Knee Cartilage Volume and Pain in Patients with Knee Osteoarthritis: A Randomized Clinical

Trial." *JAMA* 317, no. 19 (2017): 1967–75, https://doi.org/10.1001/jama.2017.5283.

7   D. S. Jevsevar. "Treatment of Osteoarthritis of the Knee: Evidence-Based Clinical Practice Guideline," 2nd edition. *Journal of American Academy of Orthopaedic Surgeons* 21, no. 9 (2013): 571–76, https://pubmed.ncbi.nlm.nih.gov/23996988/; S. L. Kolasinski, T. Neogi, M. C. Hochberg, et al. "2019 American College of Rheumatology/Arthritis Foundation Guideline for the Management of Osteoarthritis of the Hand, Hip, and Knee." *Arthritis & Rheumatology* 72, no. 2 (2020): 220–33, https://doi.org/10.1002/art.41142.

8   B. S. Ferket, Z. Feldman, J. Zhou, et al. "Impact of Total Knee Replacement Practice: Cost Effectiveness Analysis of Data from the Osteoarthritis Initiative." *British Medical Journal* 356 (2017): j1131, https://doi.org/10.1136/bmj.j1131.

9   I. Shichman, N. Askew, A. Habibi, et al. "Projections and Epidemiology of Revision Hip and Knee Arthroplasty in the United States to 2040–2060." *Arthroplasty Today* 21 (2023): 101152, https://doi.org/10.1016/j.artd.2023.101152.

10 D. F. Hamilton, C. R. Howie, R. Burnett, A. H. Simpson, and J. T. Patton. "Dealing with the Predicted Increase in Demand for Revision Total Knee Arthroplasty: Challenges, Risks and Opportunities." *Bone & Joint Journal* 97-b, no. 6 (2015): 723–28, https://doi.org/10.1302/0301-620x.97b6.35185.

11 R. A. C. Siemieniuk, I. A. Harris, T. Agoritsas, et al. "Arthroscopic Surgery for Degenerative Knee Arthritis and Meniscal Tears: A Clinical Practice Guideline." *British Journal of Sports Medicine* 52, no. 5 (2018): 313, https://doi.org/10.1136/bjsports-2017-j1982rep; J.-H. Yim, J.-K. Seon, H.-Y. Seo, et al. "A Comparative Study of Meniscectomy and Nonoperative Treatment for Degenerative Horizontal Tears of the Medial Meniscus." *American Journal of Sports Medicine* 41, no. 7 (2013): 1565–70, https://doi.org/10.1177/0363546513488518.

Chapter 4

1   S. Thomson. "Failed Back Surgery Syndrome—Definition, Epidemiology and Demographics." *British Journal of Pain* 7, no. 1 (2013): 56–59, https://doi.org/10.1177/2049463713479096.

2   T. E. Buchheit and M. Tytell. "Transfer of Molecules from Glia to Axon in the Squid May Be Mediated by Glial Vesicles." *Journal of Neurobiology* 23, no. 3 (1992): 217–30, https://doi.org/10.1002/neu .480230303.

3   S. Ahmad, R. K. Srivastava, P. Singh, U. P. Naik, and A. K. Srivastava. "Role of Extracellular Vesicles in Glia-Neuron Intercellular Communication." *Frontiers in Molecular Neuroscience* 15 (2022): 844194, https://doi.org/10.3389/fnmol.2022.844194; T. Buchheit, Y. Huh, A. Breglio, et al. "Intrathecal Administration of Conditioned Serum from Different Species Resolves Chemotherapy-Induced Neuropathic Pain in Mice via Secretory Exosomes." *Brain, Behavior, and Immunity* 111 (2023): 298–311, https://doi.org/10.1016/j.bbi.2023.04.013.

4   C. S. Evans and E. L. F. Holzbaur. "Quality Control in Neurons: Mitophagy and Other Selective Autophagy Mechanisms." *Journal of Molecular Biology* 432, no. 1 (2020): 240–60, https://doi.org/10 .1016/j.jmb.2019.06.031.

5   A. Areti, V. G. Yerra, V. Naidu, and A. Kumar. "Oxidative Stress and Nerve Damage: Role in Chemotherapy Induced Peripheral Neuropathy." *Redox Biology* 2 (2014): 289–95, https://doi.org/10 .1016/j.redox.2014.01.006.

6   C. Sommer, M. Leinders, and N. Üçeyler. "Inflammation in the Pathophysiology of Neuropathic Pain." *Pain* 159, no. 3 (2018): 595–602, https://doi.org/10.1097/j.pain.0000000000001122.

Chapter 5

1   M. C. Jensen, M. N. Brant-Zawadzki, N. Obuchowski, et al. "Magnetic Resonance Imaging of the Lumbar Spine in People Without Back Pain." *New England Journal of Medicine* 331 (1994): 69–73, https://doi.org/10.1056/nejm199407143310201.

2   J. M. Fritz, E. Lane, M. McFadden, et al. "Physical Therapy Referral from Primary Care for Acute Back Pain with Sciatica: A Randomized Controlled Trial." *Annals of Internal Medicine* 174, no. 1 (2021): 8–17, https://doi.org/10.7326/m20-4187.

3   G. A. Talebi, P. Saadat, Y. Javadian, and M. Taghipour. "Manual Therapy in the Treatment of Carpal Tunnel Syndrome in Diabetic Patients: A Randomized Clinical Trial." *Caspian Journal of Internal Medicine* 9, no. 3 (2018): 283–9, https://doi.org/10.22088 /cjim.9.3.283.

4   M. Backonja, A. Beydoun, K. R. Edwards, et al. "Gabapentin for the Symptomatic Treatment of Painful Neuropathy in Patients with Diabetes Mellitus: A Randomized Controlled Trial." *JAMA* 280, no. 21 (1998): 1831–36, https://doi.org/10.1001/jama.280.21.1831.

5   M. Rowbotham, N. Harden, B. Stacey, P. Bernstein, and L. Magnus-Miller. "Gabapentin for the Treatment of Postherpetic Neuralgia: A Randomized Controlled Trial." *JAMA* 280, no. 21 (1998): 1837–42, https://doi.org/10.1001/jama.280.21.1837.

6   N. B. Finnerup, N. Attal, S. Haroutouonian, et al. "Pharmacotherapy for Neuropathic Pain in Adults: A Systematic Review and Meta-Analysis." *Lancet Neurology* 14, no. 2 (2015): 162–73, https://doi.org/10.1016/s1474-4422(14)70251-0.

7   Finnerup et al., "Pharmacotherapy for Neuropathic Pain in Adults."

8   A. Robecchi and R. Capra. "Hydrocortisone (Compound F); First Clinical Experiments in the Field of Rheumatology." *Minerva Medica* 43, no. 98 (1952): 1259–63, https://pubmed.ncbi.nlm.nih.gov/13036739.

9   R. Chou, R. Hashimoto, J. Friedly, et al. "Epidural Corticosteroid Injections for Radiculopathy and Spinal Stenosis: A Systematic Review and Meta-Analysis." *Annals of Internal Medicine* 163, no. 5 (2015): 373–81, https://doi.org/10.7326/m15-0934.

Chapter 6

1   T. Buchheit and S. Pyati. "Prevention of Chronic Pain After Surgical Nerve Injury: Amputation and Thoracotomy." *Surgical Clinics of North America* 92, no. 2 (2012): 393–407, https://doi.org/10.1016/j.suc.2012.01.005.

2   R.-R. Ji, T. Berta, and M. Nedergaard. "Glia and Pain: Is Chronic Pain a Gliopathy?" *Pain* 154, supp. 1 (2013): S10–s28, https://doi.org/10.1016/j.pain.2013.06.022.

3   B. Liu, M. Zhang, J. Zhao, M. Zheng, and H. Yang. "Imbalance of M1/M2 Macrophages Is Linked to Severity Level of Knee Osteoarthritis." *Experimental and Therapeutic Medicine* 16 (2018): 5009–14, https://doi.org/10.3892/etm.2018.6852.

4   M. Parisien, L. V. Lima, C. Dagostino, et al. "Acute Inflammatory Response via Neutrophil Activation Protects Against the Development of Chronic Pain." *Science Translational Medicine* 14,

no. 644 (2022): eabj9954, https://doi.org/10.1126/scitranslmed
.abj9954.

5   C. R. Donnelly, C. Jiang, A. S. Andriessen, et al. "STING Controls
Nociception via Type I Interferon Signalling in Sensory Neurons."
Nature 591 (2021): 275–80, https://doi.org/10.1038/s41586-020
-03151-1.

6   T. Van de Ven, C. Donnelly, et al. Personal communication.
Publication pending.

Chapter 7

1   A. E. Rumora, G. LoGrasso, J. M. Hayes, et al. "The Divergent Roles
of Dietary Saturated and Monounsaturated Fatty Acids on Nerve
Function in Murine Models of Obesity." *Journal of Neuroscience* 39,
no. 19 (2019): 3770–81, https://doi.org/10.1523/jneurosci.3173
-18.2019.

2   K. R. Baker, N. R. Matthan, A. H. Lichtenstein, et al. "Association of
Plasma n-6 and n-3 Polyunsaturated Fatty Acids with Synovitis in
the Knee: The MOST Study." *Osteoarthritis and Cartilage* 20, no. 5
(2012): 382–87, https://doi.org/10.1016/j.joca.2012.01.021.

3   J. T. Boyd, P. M. LoCoco, A. R. Furr, et al. "Elevated Dietary ⍵-6
Polyunsaturated Fatty Acids Induce Reversible Peripheral Nerve
Dysfunction That Exacerbates Comorbid Pain Conditions." *Nature
Metabolism* 3 (2021): 762–73, https://doi.org/10.1038/s42255
-021-00410-x.

4   W. Deng, Z. Yi, E. Yin, R. Lu, H. You, and X. Yuan. "Effect of
Omega-3 Polyunsaturated Fatty Acids Supplementation for Patients
with Osteoarthritis: A Meta-Analysis." *Journal of Orthopaedic
Surgery and Research* 18, no. 381 (2023): https://doi.org
/10.1186/s13018-023-03855-w.

5   Baker et al. "Association of Plasma n-6 and n-3 Polyunsaturated
Fatty Acids with Synovitis in the Knee."

6   Boyd et al. "Elevated Dietary ⍵-6 Polyunsaturated Fatty Acids
Induce Reversible Peripheral Nerve Dysfunction That Exacerbates
Comorbid Pain Conditions."

7   Z. Ghoreishi, Z. A. Esfahani, A. Djazayeri, et al. "Omega-3 Fatty
Acids Are Protective Against Paclitaxel-Induced Peripheral
Neuropathy: A Randomized Double-Blind Placebo Controlled

Trial." *BMC Cancer* 12, no. 355 (2012): https://doi.org/10.1186 /1471-2407-12-355.

8 C. E. Ramsden, D. Zamora, K. R. Faurot, et al. "Dietary Alteration of n-3 and n-6 Fatty Acids for Headache Reduction in Adults with Migraine: Randomized Controlled Trial." *BMJ* 374, no. 1448 (2021): https://doi.org/10.1136/bmj.n1448.

9 C. Santa-María, S. López-Enriquez, S. Montserrat-de la Paz, et al. "Update on Anti-Inflammatory Molecular Mechanisms Induced by Oleic Acid." *Nutrients* 15, no. 1 (2023): https://doi.org/10.3390 /nu15010224.

10 Rumora et al. "The Divergent Roles of Dietary Saturated and Monounsaturated Fatty Acids on Nerve Function in Murine Models of Obesity."

11 R. Estruch, E. Ros, J. Salas-Salvadó, et al. "Primary Prevention of Cardiovascular Disease with a Mediterranean Diet Supplemented with Extra-Virgin Olive Oil or Nuts." *New England Journal of Medicine* 378, no. 25 (2018): e34, https://doi.org/10.1056/NEJMoa1800389.

12 M. Barchitta, A. Maugeri, G. Favara, et al. "Nutrition and Wound Healing: An Overview Focusing on the Beneficial Effects of Curcumin." *International Journal of Molecular Sciences* 20, no. 5 (2019): 1119, https://doi.org/10.3390/ijms20051119.

13 N. Veronese, L. La Tegola, G. Crepaldi, S. Maggi, D. Rogoli, and G. Guglielmi. "The Association Between the Mediterranean Diet and Magnetic Resonance Parameters for Knee Osteoarthritis: Data from the Osteoarthritis Initiative." *Clinical Rheumatology* 37 (2018): 2187–93, https://doi.org/10.1007/s10067-018-4075-5.

Chapter 8

1 C. Bernard, A. Zavoriti, Q. Pucelle, B. Chazaud, and J. Gondin. "Role of Macrophages During Skeletal Muscle Regeneration and Hypertrophy-Implications for Immunomodulatory Strategies." *Physiological Reports* 10, no. 19 (2022): e15480, https://doi.org/10 .14814/phy2.15480.

2 T. M. Kistner, B. K. Pedersen, and D. E. Lieberman. "Interleukin 6 as an Energy Allocator in Muscle Tissue." *Nature Metabolism* 4 (2022): 170–79, https://doi.org/10.1038/s42255-022-00538-4.

3 J. K. Smith. "Exercise as an Adjuvant to Cartilage Regeneration Therapy." *International Journal of Molecular Sciences* 21, no. 24 (2020): https://doi.org/10.3390/ijms21249471.

4 H. Alexanderson. "Exercise Effects in Patients with Adult Idiopathic Inflammatory Myopathies." *Current Opinion in Rheumatology* 21, no. 2 (2009): 158–63, https://doi.org/10.1097/BOR.0b013e328324e700.

5 H. Alexanderson. "Exercise Effects in Patients with Adult Idiopathic Inflammatory Myopathies."

6 J. F. Markworth, L. D. Vella, V. C. Figueiredo, and D. Cameron-Smith. "Ibuprofen Treatment Blunts Early Translational Signaling Responses in Human Skeletal Muscle Following Resistance Exercise." *Journal of Applied Physiology* 117, no. 1 (2014): 20–28, https://doi.org/10.1152/japplphysiol.01299.2013.

7 C. Bernard, A. Zavoriti, Q. Pucelle, B. Chazaud, and J. Gondin. "Role of Macrophages During Skeletal Muscle Regeneration and Hypertrophy-Implications for Immunomodulatory Strategies." *Physiological Reports* 10, no. 19 (2022): e15480, https://doi.org/10.14814/phy2.15480.

8 S. Hinterwimmer, M. Krammer, M. Krötz, et al. "Cartilage Atrophy in the Knees of Patients After Seven Weeks of Partial Load Bearing." *Arthritis & Rheumatology* 50, no. 8 (2004): 2516–20, https://doi.org/10.1002/art.20378.

9 C. Y. Zeng, Z. R. Zhang, Z. M. Tang, and F. Z. Hua. "Benefits and Mechanisms of Exercise Training for Knee Osteoarthritis." *Frontiers in Physiology* 12 (2021): 794062, https://doi.org/10.3389/fphys.2021.794062.

10 S. R. O'Connor, M. A. Tully, B. Ryan, et al. "Walking Exercise for Chronic Musculoskeletal Pain: Systematic Review and Meta-Analysis." *Archives of Physical Medicine and Rehabilitation* 96, no. 4 (2015): 724–34.E23, https://doi.org/10.1016/j.apmr.2014.12.003.

11 G. H. Lo, S. Vinod, M. J. Richard, et al. "Association Between Walking for Exercise and Symptomatic and Structural Progression in Individuals with Knee Osteoarthritis: Data from the Osteoarthritis Initiative Cohort." *Arthritis & Rheumatology* 74, no. 10 (2022): 1660–67, https://doi.org/10.1002/art.42241.

12 J. Dhillon, M. J. Kraeutler, J. W. Belk, et al. "Effects of Running on the Development of Knee Osteoarthritis: An Updated Systematic

Review at Short-Term Follow-Up." *Orthopaedic Journal of Sports Medicine* 11, no. 3 (2023). https://doi.org/10.1177 /23259671231152900.

13   C. Cheung, J. F. Wyman, B. Resnick, and K. Savik. "Yoga for Managing Knee Osteoarthritis in Older Women: A Pilot Randomized Controlled Trial." *BMC Complementary Medicine and Therapies* 14, no. 160 (2014): https://doi.org/10.1186/1472 -6882-14-160.

14   L. Hu, Y. Wang, X. Liu, et al. "Tai Chi Exercise Can Ameliorate Physical and Mental Health of Patients with Knee Osteoarthritis: Systematic Review and Meta-Analysis." *Clinical Rehabilitation* 35, no. 1 (2020): 64–79, https://doi.org/10.1177/0269215520954343.

15   L. Hu, Y. Wang, X. Liu, et al. "Tai Chi Exercise Can Ameliorate Physical and Mental Health of Patients with Knee Osteoarthritis: Systematic Review and Meta-Analysis."

Chapter 9

1   J. M. Fritz, E. Lane, M. McFadden, et al. "Physical Therapy Referral from Primary Care for Acute Back Pain with Sciatica: A Randomized Controlled Trial." *Annals of Internal Medicine* 174, no. 1 (2021): 8–17, https://doi.org/10.7326/m20-4187; H. B. Albert and C. Manniche. "The Efficacy of Systematic Active Conservative Treatment for Patients with Severe Sciatica: A Single-Blind, Randomized, Clinical, Controlled Trial." *Spine* 37, no. 7 (2012): 531–42, https://doi.org/10.1097/BRS.0b013e31821ace7f; D. Kernc, V. Strojnik, and R. Vengust. "Early Initiation of a Strength Training Based Rehabilitation After Lumbar Spine Fusion Improves Core Muscle Strength: A Randomized Controlled Trial." *Journal of Orthopaedic Surgery and Research* 13, 151 (2018), https://doi.org/10 .1186/s13018-018-0853-7.

2   F. Streckmann, E. M. Zopf, H. C. Lehmann, et al. "Exercise Intervention Studies in Patients with Peripheral Neuropathy: A Systematic Review." *Sports Medicine* 44 (2014): 1289–304, https://doi.org/10.1007/s40279-014-0207-5.

3   S. Dixit, A. Maiya, and B. A. Shastry. "Effects of Aerobic Exercise on Vibration Perception Threshold in Type 2 Diabetic Peripheral Neuropathy Population Using 3-sites Method: Single-Blind Randomized Controlled Trial." *Alternative Therapies in Health and*

Medicine 25, no. 2 (2019): 36–41, https://pubmed.ncbi.nlm.nih.gov /30990792.

4 I. R. Kleckner, C. Kamen, J. S. Gewandter, et al. "Effects of Exercise During Chemotherapy on Chemotherapy-Induced Peripheral Neuropathy: A Multicenter, Randomized Controlled Trial." *Supportive Care in Cancer* 26 (2018): 1019–28, https://doi.org /10.1007/s00520-017-4013-0.

5 S. Balducci, G. Iacobellis, L. Parisi, et al. "Exercise Training Can Modify the Natural History of Diabetic Peripheral Neuropathy." *Journal of Diabetes and Its Complications* 20, no. 4 (2006): 216–23, https://doi.org/10.1016/j.jdiacomp.2005.07.005.

6 P. M. Kluding, M. Pasnoor, R. Singh, et al. "The Effect of Exercise on Neuropathic Symptoms, Nerve Function, and Cutaneous Innervation in People with Diabetic Peripheral Neuropathy." *Journal of Diabetes and Its Complications* 26, no. 5 (2012): 424–29, https://doi.org/10.1016/j.jdiacomp.2012.05.007.

7 J. R. Singleton, R. L. Marcus, J. E. Jackson, et al. "Exercise Increases Cutaneous Nerve Density in Diabetic Patients Without Neuropathy." *Annals of Clinical and Translational Neurology* 1, no. 10 (2014): 844–49, https://doi.org/10.1002/acn3.125.

8 R. Kalluri and V. S. LeBleu. "The Biology, Function, and Biomedical Applications of Exosomes." *Science* 367, no. 6478 (2020): https://doi.org/10.1126/science.aau6977.

9 J. P. Nederveen, G. Warnier, A. Di Carlo, M. I. Nilsson, and M. A. Tarnopolsky. "Extracellular Vesicles and Exosomes: Insights from Exercise Science." *Frontiers in Physiology* 11, 604274 (2020): https://doi.org/10.3389/fphys.2020.604274.

10 H. Song, J. Zhao, J. Cheng, et al. "Extracellular Vesicles in Chondrogenesis and Cartilage Regeneration." *Journal of Cellular and Molecular Medicine* 25, no. 11 (2021): 4883–92, https://doi.org/10.1111/jcmm.16290.

11 T. Buchheit, Y. Huh, A. Breglio, et al. "Intrathecal Administration of Conditioned Serum from Different Species Resolves Chemotherapy-Induced Neuropathic Pain in Mice via Secretory Exosomes." *Brain, Behavior, and Immuity* 111 (2023): 298–311, https://doi.org/10.1016/j.bbi.2023.04.013.

12 T. Buchheit, et al. "Intrathecal Administration of Conditioned Serum from Different Species Resolves Chemotherapy-Induced Neuropathic Pain in Mice via Secretory Exosomes."

Chapter 10

1   O. Gabay and C. Sanchez. "Epigenetics, Sirtuins and Osteoarthritis. *Joint Bone Spine* 79, no. 6 (2012): 570–73, https://doi.org/10.1016/j .jbspin.2012.04.005.

2   T. Buchheit, T., Van de Ven, and A. Shaw. "Epigenetics and the Transition from Acute to Chronic Pain. *Pain Med* 13, no. 11 (2012): 1474–90, https://doi.org/10.1111/j.1526-4637.2012.01488.x.

3   B. Sowikowski, W. Owecki, J. Jeske, et al. "Epigenetics and the Neurodegenerative Process." *Epigenomics* 16, no. 7 (2024): 473–91, https://doi.org/10.2217/epi-2023-0416.

4   J.-H. Yang, M. Hayano, P. T. Griffin, et al. "Loss of Epigenetic Information as a Cause of Mammalian Aging." *Cell* 186, no. 2 (2023): 305–26.E327, https://doi.org/10.1016/j.cell.2022.12.027.

5   R. A. H. van de Ven, D. Santos, and M. C. Haigis. "Mitochondrial Sirtuins and Molecular Mechanisms of Aging." *Trends Molecular Medicine* 23, no. 4 (2017): 320–31, https://doi.org/10.1016/j.molmed .2017.02.005.

6   O. Gabay and C. Sanchez. "Epigenetics, Sirtuins and Osteoarthritis." *Joint Bone Spine.*

7   C. G. Juan, K. B. Matchett, and G. W. Davison. "A Systematic Review and Meta-Analysis of the SIRT1 Response to Exercise." *Scientific Reports* 13, art. no. 14752 (2023): https://doi.org/10.1038 /s41598-023-38843-x.

8   S. Horvath and K. Raj. "DNA Methylation-Based Biomarkers and the Epigenetic Clock Theory of Ageing." *Nature Reviews Genetics* 19 (2018): 371–84, https://doi.org/10.1038/s41576-018-0004-3.

9   K. N. Fitzgerald, R. Hodges, D. Hanes, et al. "Potential Reversal of Epigenetic Age Using a Diet and Lifestyle Intervention: A Pilot Randomized Clinical Trial." *Aging* 13, no. 7: (2021): 9419–32, https://doi.org/10.18632/aging.202913.

10 Y. Zhang, S. Li, P. Jin, et al. "Dual Functions of microRNA-17 in Maintaining Cartilage Homeostasis and Protection Against Osteoarthritis." *Nature Communications* 13, art. no. 2447 (2022): https://doi.org/10.1038/s41467-022-30119-8.

11 R. López-Leal, F. Díaz-Viraqué, R. J. Catalán, et al. "Schwann Cell Reprogramming into Repair Cells Increases miRNA-21 Expression in Exosomes Promoting Axonal Growth." *Journal of Cell Science* 133, no. 12 (2020): https://doi.org/10.1242/jcs.239004.

12 S. Cosenza, M. Ruiz, K. Toupet, C. Jorgensen, and D. Noël. "Mesenchymal Stem Cells Derived Exosomes and Microparticles Protect Cartilage and Bone from Degradation in Osteoarthritis." *Scientific Reports* 7, art. no. 16214 (2017): https://doi.org/10.1038/s41598-017-15376-8.

13 M. S. Namini, F. Daneshimehr, N. Beheshtizadeh, et al. "Cell-Free Therapy Based on Extracellular Vesicles: A Promising Therapeutic Strategy for Peripheral Nerve Injury." *Stem Cell Research & Therapy* 14, art. no. 254 (2023): https://doi.org/10.1186/s13287-023-03467-5.

14 C. Loussouarn, Y. M. Pers, C. Bony, C. Jorgensen, and D. Noël. "Mesenchymal Stromal Cell-Derived Extracellular Vesicles Regulate the Mitochondrial Metabolism via Transfer of miRNAs." *Frontiers in Immunology* 12, art. no. 623973 (2021): https://doi.org/10.3389/fimmu.2021.623973.

15 V. D. Nair, Y. Ge, S. Li, H. Pincas, et al. "Sedentary and Trained Older Men Have Distinct Circulating Exosomal microRNA Profiles at Baseline and in Response to Acute Exercise." *Frontiers in Physiology* 11, art. no. 605 (2020): https://doi.org/10.3389/fphys.2020.00605.

Chapter 11

1 D. R. Knighton, K. F. Ciresi, V. D. Fiegel, L. L. Austin, and E. L. Butler. "Classification and Treatment of Chronic Nonhealing Wounds. Successful Treatment with Autologous Platelet-Derived Wound Healing Factors (PDWHF)." *Annals of Surgery* 204, no. 3 (1986): 322–30, https://doi.org/10.1097/00000658-198609000-00011.

2 R. E. Marx, E. R. Carlson, R. M. Eichstaedt, et al. "Platelet-Rich Plasma: Growth Factor Enhancement for Bone Grafts." *Oral Surgery, Oral Medicine, Oral Pathology* 85, no. 6 (1998): 638–46, https://doi.org/10.1016/s1079-2104(98)90029-4.

3 E. Kon, R. Buda, G. Filardo, et al. "Platelet-Rich Plasma: Intra-Articular Knee Injections Produced Favorable Results on Degenerative Cartilage Lesions." *Knee Surgery Sports Traumatology Arthroscopy* 18, no. 4 (2010): 472–79, https://doi.org/10.1007/s00167-009-0940-8; A. Mishra and T. Pavelko. "Treatment of Chronic Elbow Tendinosis with Buffered Platelet-Rich Plasma." *American Journal of Sports Medicine* 34, no. 11 (2006): 1774–78, https://doi.org/10.1177/0363546506288850.

4   M. C. Hochberg, A. Guermazi, H. Guehring, et al. "Effect of Intra-Articular Sprifermin vs Placebo on Femorotibial Joint Cartilage Thickness in Patients With Osteoarthritis: The FORWARD Randomized Clinical Trial." *JAMA* 322, no. 14 (2019): 1360–70, https://doi.org/10.1001/jama.2019.14735.

5   J.-P. Pujol, C. Chadjichristos, F. Legendre, et al. "Interleukin-1 and Transforming Growth Factor-ß 1 as Crucial Factors in Osteoarthritic Cartilage Metabolism." *Connective Tissue Research* 49 (2009): 293–97, https://doi.org/10.1080/03008200802148355.

6   H. Singh, D. M. Knapik, E. M. Polce, et al. "Relative Efficacy of Intra-Articular Injections in the Treatment of Knee Osteoarthritis: A Systematic Review and Network Meta-Analysis." *American Journal of Sports Medicine* 50, no. 11 (2021): 3635465211029659, https://doi.org/10.1177/03635465211029659.

7   J. L. Hudgens, K. B. Sugg, J. A. Grekin, et al. "Platelet-Rich Plasma Activates Proinflammatory Signaling Pathways and Induces Oxidative Stress in Tendon Fibroblasts." *American Journal of Sports Medicine* 44, no. 8 (2016): 1931–40, https://doi.org/10.1177/0363546516637176; H. J. Braun, H. J. Kim, C. R. Chu, and J. L. Dragoo. "The Effect of Platelet-Rich Plasma Formulations and Blood Products on Human Synoviocytes: Implications for Intra-Articular Injury and Therapy." *American Journal of Sports Medicine* 42, no. 5 (2014): 1204–10, https://doi.org/10.1177/0363546514525593.

8   K. L. Bennell, K. L. Paterson, B. R. Metcalf, et al. "Effect of Intra-articular Platelet-Rich Plasma vs Placebo Injection on Pain and Medial Tibial Cartilage Volume in Patients with Knee Osteoarthritis: The RESTORE Randomized Clinical Trial." *JAMA* 326, no. 20 (2021): 2021–30, https://doi.org/10.1001/jama.2021.19415.

9   S. Wang, X. Liu, and Y. Wang. "Evaluation of Platelet-Rich Plasma Therapy for Peripheral Nerve Regeneration: A Critical Review of Literature." *Frontiers in Bioengingeering and Biotechnology* 10 (2022): 808248, https://doi.org/10.3389/fbioe.2022.808248.

10 K. R. Ko, J. Lee, D. Lee, B. Nho, and S. Kim. "Hepatocyte Growth Factor (HGF) Promotes Peripheral Nerve Regeneration by Activating Repair Schwann Cells." *Scientific Reports* 8, art. no. 8316 (2018), https://doi.org/10.1038/s41598-018-26704-x.

11 T. Buchheit, Y. Huh, W. Maixner, J. Cheng, and R.-R. Ji. "Neuroimmune Modulation of Pain and Regenerative Pain

Medicine." *Journal of Clinical Investigation* 130, no. 5 (2020): 2164–76, https://doi.org/10.1172/JCI134439.

12 C. Dong, Y. Sun, Y. Qi, et al. "Effect of Platelet-Rich Plasma Injection on Mild or Moderate Carpal Tunnel Syndrome: An Updated Systematic Review and Meta-Analysis of Randomized Controlled Trials." *BioMed Research International 2020*, 5089378 (2020): https://doi.org/10.1155/2020/5089378.

13 M. Hassanien, A. Elawamy, E. Z. Kamel, et al. "Perineural Platelet-Rich Plasma for Diabetic Neuropathic Pain, Could It Make a Difference?" *Pain Medicine* 21, no. 4 (2020): 757–65, https://doi.org/10.1093/pm/pnz140.

14 J. Zhao, H. Huang, G. Liang, L.-F. Zeng, W. Yang, and J. Liu. "Effects and Safety of the Combination of Platelet-Rich Plasma (PRP) and Hyaluronic Acid (HA) in the Treatment of Knee Osteoarthritis: A Systematic Review and Meta-Analysis." *BMC Musculoskeletal Disorders* 21, art. no. 224 (2020): https://doi.org/10.1186/s12891-020-03262-w.

Chapter 12

1 A. I. Caplan. "Mesenchymal Stem Cells." *Journal of Orthopaedic Research* 9, no. 5 (1991): 641–50, https://doi.org/10.1002/jor.1100090504.

2 J. M. Murphy, D. J. Fink, E. B. Hunziker, and F. P. Barry. "Stem Cell Therapy in a Caprine Model of Osteoarthritis." *Arthritis & Rheumatology* 48, no. 12 (2003): 3464–74, https://doi.org/10.1002/art.11365.

3 C. J. Centeno, D. Busse, J. Kisiday, C. Keohan, M. Freeman, and D. Karli. "Increased Knee Cartilage Volume in Degenerative Joint Disease Using Percutaneously Implanted, Autologous Mesenchymal Stem Cells." *Pain Physician* 11, no. 3 (2008): 343–53, https://www.painphysicianjournal.com/current/pdf?article=OTk3&journal=43.

4 A. Vega, M. A. Martin-Ferrero, F. Del Canto, et al. "Treatment of Knee Osteoarthritis with Allogeneic Bone Marrow Mesenchymal Stem Cells." *Transplantation* 99, no. 8 (2015): 1681–90, https://doi.org/10.1097/tp.0000000000000678.

5 M. Satué, C. Schüler, N. Ginner, and R. G. Erben. "Intra-Articularly Injected Mesenchymal Stem Cells Promote Cartilage Regeneration, But Do Not Permanently Engraft in Distant Organs." *Scientific*

Report 9, art. no. 10153 (2019): https://doi.org/10.1038/s41598
-019-46554-5.

6   Y. G. Koh, Y. L. Choi, O. R. Kwon, and Y. S. Kim." Second-Look
Arthroscopic Evaluation of Cartilage Lesions After Mesenchymal
Stem Cell Implantation in Osteoarthritic Knees." *American Journal
of Sports Medicine* 42, no. 7 (2014): 1628–3, https://doi.org/10.1177
/0363546514529641.

7   J. Matas, M. Orrego, D. Amenabar, et al. "Umbilical Cord-Derived
Mesenchymal Stromal Cells (MSCs) for Knee Osteoarthritis:
Repeated MSC Dosing Is Superior to a Single MSC Dose and to
Hyaluronic Acid in a Controlled Randomized Phase I/II Trial."
Stem Cells Translational Medicine 8, no. 3 (2019): 215–24,
https://doi.org/10.1002/sctm.18-0053.

8   S. H. Kim, Y. P. Djaja, Y.-B. Park, et al. "Intra-Articular Injection
of Culture-Expanded Mesenchymal Stem Cells Without Adjuvant
Surgery in Knee Osteoarthritis: A Systematic Review and Meta-
analysis." *American Journal of Sports Medicine* 48, no. 7 (2020):
2839–49, https://doi.org/10.1177/0363546519892278.

9   R. A. Charo and D. Sipp." Rejuvenating Regenerative Medicine
Regulation." *New England Journal of Medicine* 378, no. 6 (2018):
504–05, https://doi.org/10.1056/nejmp1715736; K. P. Hartnett,
K. M. Powell, D. Rankin, et al. "Investigation of Bacterial Infections
Among Patients Treated with Umbilical Cord Blood-Derived
Products Marketed as Stem Cell Therapies." *JAMA Network Open* 4,
no. 10 (2021): e2128615, https://doi.org/10.1001
/jamanetworkopen.2021.28615

10 S. H. S. Tan, Y. T. Kwan, W. J. Neo, et al. "Intra-Articular Injections
of Mesenchymal Stem Cells Without Adjuvant Therapies for Knee
Osteoarthritis: A Systematic Review and Meta-Analysis." *American
Journal of Sports Medicine* 49, no. 11 (2021): 3113–24, https://doi.org
/10.1177/0363546520981704.

11 K. Mautner, M. Gottschalk, S. D. Boden, et al. "Cell-Based Versus
Corticosteroid Injections for Knee Pain in Osteoarthritis: A
Randomized Phase 3 Trial." *Nature Medicine* 29 (2023): 3120–26,
https://doi.org/10.1038/s41591-023-02632-w.

12 A. W. Anz, R. Hubbard, N. K. Rendos, et al. "Bone Marrow
Aspirate Concentrate Is Equivalent to Platelet-Rich Plasma for
the Treatment of Knee Osteoarthritis at 1 Year: A Prospective,

Randomized Trial." *Orthopaedic Journal of Sports Medicine* 8, no. 2 (2020): https://doi.org/10.1177/2325967119900958.

13 A. H. Gomoll, J. Farr, B. J. Cole, et al. "Safety and Efficacy of an Amniotic Suspension Allograft Injection Over 12 Months in a Single-Blinded, Randomized Controlled Trial for Symptomatic Osteoarthritis of the Knee." *Journal of Arthroscopy and Related Surgery* 37, no. 7 (2021): 2246–57, https://doi.org/10.1016/j.arthro .2021.02.044.

14 A. I. Caplan. "What's in a Name?" *Tissue Engineering Part A* 16, no. 8 (2010): 2415–17, https://doi.org/10.1089/ten.TEA.2010.0216.

Chapter 13

1 G. Chen, C. K. Park, R. G. Xie, and R. R. Ji. "Intrathecal Bone Marrow Stromal Cells Inhibit Neuropathic Pain via TGF-Beta Secretion." *Journal of Clinical Investigation* 125, no. 8 (2015): 3226–40, https://doi.org/10.1172/JCI80883.

2 S. R. Cho, Y. R. Kim, H.-S. Kang, et al. "Functional Recovery After the Transplantation of Neurally Differentiated Mesenchymal Stem Cells Derived from Bone Marrow in a Rat Model of Spinal Cord Injury." *Cell Transplantation* 18, no. 12 (2009): 1359–68, https://doi.org /10.3727/096368909x475329.

3 L. Liu, Z. Hua, J. Shen, et al. "Comparative Efficacy of Multiple Variables of Mesenchymal Stem Cell Transplantation for the Treatment of Neuropathic Pain in Rats." *Military Medicine* 182, supp. 1 (2017): 175–84, https://doi.org/10.7205/milmed-d-16 -00096

4 S. F. H. de Witte, F. Luk, J. M. Sierra Parraga, et al. "Immunomodulation by Therapeutic Mesenchymal Stromal Cells (MSC) Is Triggered Through Phagocytosis of MSC by Monocytic Cells." *Stem Cells* 36, no. 4 (2018): 602–15, https://doi.org/10.1002 /stem.2779; W. Guo, S. Imai, J.-L. Yang, et al. "In Vivo Immune Interactions of Multipotent Stromal Cells Underlie Their Long-Lasting Pain-Relieving Effect." *Scientific Reports* 7, art. no. 10107 (2017): https://doi.org/10.1038/s41598-017-10251-y.

5 W. Guo, S. Imai, J.-L. Yang, et al. "In Vivo Immune Interactions of Multipotent Stromal Cells Underlie Their Long-Lasting Pain-Relieving Effect." *Scientific Reports* 7, art. no. 10107 (2017), https://doi .org/10.1038/s41598-017-10251-y.

6   S. W. Mitchell. *Injuries of Nerves and Their Consequences* (J. B. Lippincott, 1872).

7   J. David Clark, V. L. Tawfik, M. Tajerian, and W. S. Kingery. "Autoinflammatory and Autoimmune Contributions to Complex Regional Pain Syndrome." *Molecular Pain* 14, art. no. 1744806918799127 (2018): https://doi.org/10.1177 /1744806918799127.

8   M. Zavatti, F. Beretti, F. Casciaro, E. Bertucci, and T. Maraldi. "Comparison of the Therapeutic Effect of Amniotic Fluid Stem Cells and Their Exosomes on Monoiodoacetate-Induced Animal Model of Osteoarthritis." *BioFactors* 46 (2020): 106–17, https://doi .org/10.1002/biof.1576.

Chapter 14

1   P. Wehling, S. J. Cleveland, K. Heininger, K P. Schulitz, J. Reinecke, and C. H. Evans. "Neurophysiologic Changes in Lumbar Nerve Root Inflammation in the Rat After Treatment with Cytokine Inhibitors." *Spine* 21, no. 8 (1996): 931–35, https://doi.org/10.1097 /00007632-199604150-00005.

2   H. Meijer, J. Reinecke, C. Becker, G. Tholen, and P. Wehling, P. "The Production of Anti-Inflammatory Cytokines in Whole Blood by Physico-Chemical Induction." *Inflammation Research* 52 (2003): 404–07, https://doi.org/10.1007/s00011-003-1197-1.

3   P. R. Wehling and H. Meijer. "Injections with Interleukin-1-Receptor-Antagonist (IRAP) in Lumbar Radicular Compression: Pathophysiologic Background, Safety, and Clinical Results," presented at the Congress of the International Society for the Study of the Lumbar Spine, Brussels, Belgium, 1998.

4   C. Becker, S. Heidersdorf, S. Drewlo, S. Z. de Rodriguez, J. Krämer, and R. E. Willburger. "Efficacy of Epidural Perineural Injections With Autologous Conditioned Serum for Lumbar Radicular Compression." *Spine* 32, no. 17 (2007): 1803–08, https://doi.org/10 .1097/brs.0b013e3181076514.

5   A. W. A. Baltzer, C. Moser, S. A. Jansen, and R. Krauspe. "Autologous Conditioned Serum (Orthokine) Is an Effective Treatment for Knee Osteoarthritis." *Osteoarthritis Cartilage* 17, no. 2 (2009): 152–60, https://doi.org/10.1016/j.joca.2008.06.014.

6   A. W. A. Baltzer, M. S. Ostapczuk, D. Stosch, F. Seidel, and M. Granrath. "A New Treatment for Hip Osteoarthritis: Clinical

Evidence for the Efficacy of Autologous Conditioned Serum." *Orthopedic Reviews* 5, no. 2 (2013): e13, https://doi.org/10.4081/or .2013.e13.

7 N. Damjanov, B. Barac, J. Colic, V. Stevanovic, A. Zekovic, and G. Tulic. "The Efficacy and Safety of Autologous Conditioned Serum (ACS) Injections Compared with Betamethasone and Placebo Injections in the Treatment of Chronic Shoulder Joint Pain Due to Supraspinatus Tendinopathy: A Prospective, Randomized, Double-Blind, Controlled Study." *Medical Ultrasonography* 20, no. 3 (2018): 335–41, https://doi.org/10.11152/mu-1495.

8 X. Chevalier, P. Goupille, A. D. Beaulieu, et al. "Intraarticular Injection of Anakinra in Osteoarthritis of the Knee: A Multicenter, Randomized, Double-Blind, Placebo-Controlled Study." *Arthritis & Rheumatism* 61, no. 3 (2009): 344–52: https://doi.org/10.1002/art .24096.

9 T. Buchheit, Y. Huh, A. Breglio, et al. "Intrathecal Administration of Conditioned Serum from Different Species Resolves Chemotherapy-Induced Neuropathic Pain in Mice via Secretory Exosomes." *Brain, Behavior, and Immununity* 111 (2023): 298–311, https://doi.org/10.1016/j.bbi.2023.04.013.

10 G. Mao, Z. Zhang, S. Hu, et al. "Exosomes Derived from miR-92a-3p-Overexpressing Human Mesenchymal Stem Cells Enhance Chondrogenesis and Suppress Cartilage Degradation via Targeting WNT5A." *Stem Cell Research & Therapy* 9, art. no. 247 (2018): https://doi.org/10.1186/s13287-018-1004-0.

11 B. Fan, C. Li, A. Szalad, et al. "Mesenchymal Stromal Cell-Derived Exosomes Ameliorate Peripheral Neuropathy in a Mouse Model of Diabetes." *Diabetologia* 63 (2020): 431–43, https://doi.org/10.1007 /s00125-019-05043-0.

Chapter 15

1 H. Bansal, J. Leon, J. L. Pont, et al. "Platelet-Rich Plasma (PRP) in Osteoarthritis (OA) Knee: Correct Dose Critical for Long Term Clinical Efficacy. *Scientific Reports* 11, art. no. 3971 (2021): https://doi .org/10.1038/s41598-021-83025-2; A. W. Anz, R. Hubbard, N. K. Rendos, et al. "Bone Marrow Aspirate Concentrate Is Equivalent to Platelet-Rich Plasma for the Treatment of Knee Osteoarthritis at 1 Year: A Prospective, Randomized Trial." *Orthopaedic Journal of Sports Medicine* 8, no. 2 (2020): https://doi.org/10.1177

/2325967119900958; K. L. Bennell, K. L. Paterson, B. R. Metcalf, et al. "Effect of Intra-Articular Platelet-Rich Plasma vs Placebo Injection on Pain and Medial Tibial Cartilage Volume in Patients with Knee Osteoarthritis: The RESTORE Randomized Clinical Trial." *JAMA* 326, no. 20 (2021): 2021–30, https://doi.org/10.1001/jama.2021.19415; T. Buchheit, C. Hunt, J. Eldrige, Y. Eshraghi, and D. Souza. "Product Characteristics Should Be Reported in All Biological Therapy Publications." *Regional Anesthesia & Pain Medicine* 47 (2022): 449, https://doi.org/10.1136/rapm-2022-103557.

2   A. W. Anz, R. Hubbard, N. K. Rendos, et al. "Bone Marrow Aspirate Concentrate Is Equivalent to Platelet-Rich Plasma for the Treatment of Knee Osteoarthritis at 1 Year: A Prospective, Randomized Trial." *Orthopaedic Journal of Sports Medicine* 8, no. 2 (2020): https://doi.org/10.1177/2325967119900958.

Index

Note: Page numbers followed by *f* indicate a figure.